RECENT ADVANCES IN INFECTIVE ENDOCARDITIS

Edited by **Steven W. Kerrigan**

Recent Advances in Infective Endocarditis
http://dx.doi.org/10.5772/46221
Edited by Steven W. Kerrigan

Contributors

Ozlem Sahin, Steve W. W. Kerrigan, Dorothea Tilley, Inmaculada Tomás-Carmona, Maximiliano Álvarez-Fernández, Yongping Wang, Aifeng Wang, Nicholas Kang

Published by InTech

Janeza Trdine 9, 51000 Rijeka, Croatia

Publishing Process Manager Ana Pantar
Technical Editor InTech DTP team
Cover InTech Design team

Additional hard copies can be obtained from orders@intechopen.com

Recent Advances in Infective Endocarditis, Edited by Steven W. Kerrigan
p. cm.
ISBN 978-953-51-1169-6

For EU product safety concerns:
IN TECH d.o.o., Prolaz Marije Krucifikse Kozulić 3, 51000 Rijeka, Croatia,
info@intechopen.com or visit our website at intechopen.com.

Meet the editor

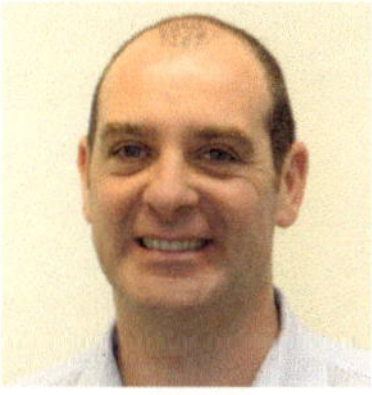

Dr. Steven W. Kerrigan received a PhD in characterising platelet-bacterial interactions from the Department of Clinical Pharmacology in the Royal College of Surgeons in Ireland in 2001. Following postdoctoral research in the USA, Dr. Kerrigan was awarded the prestigious Health Research Board of Ireland Postdoctoral Fellowship from which he set-up the internationally recognised Cardiovascular Infection Research Group in the Royal College of Surgeons in Ireland. Dr. Kerrigan is now a recognised world leader in Infective Endocarditis and has published many papers in high impact journals which make a significant contribution to our understanding this complex disease.

Contents

Preface

Infective Endocarditis is considered to be the fourth leading cause of life threatening infectious disease, and is associated with significant morbidity and mortality. It typically develops in individuals with an underlying cardiac defect, and usually occurs in close proximity to lesions subjected to hemodynamic disturbance. These lesions have the ability to generate turbulent blood flow, which in turn can damage the endothelial surface, exposing the subendothelial matrix. This area becomes highly thrombogenic, leading to platelet deposition and the formation of a fibrin network. This sterile platelet fibrin nidus, in turn, recruits bacteria from either a distal source or from a focal infection resulting from transient bacteraemia. Finally, secondary accumulation of platelets encase the bacteria forming a septic thrombus rendering them safe from immune attack. Thrombus formation can lead to aortic valve leaflet perforation that can manifest itself as acute congestive heart failure.

Treatment of infective endocarditis usually requires a multidisciplinary approach involving specialists in infectious disease, cardiologists and cardiac surgeons. Current treatment regimes consist of aggressive prolonged antibiotic therapy, frequently combined with surgery. Prolonged antibiotic use is often less than successful as 40% of patients relapse within 2 months of finishing clinically effective therapy. Furthermore, prolonged exposure to antibiotics leads to a greater risk of adding to the global problem of multiple antibiotic resistant strains of bacteria. Surgery is a costly and risky alternative, however necessary in up to 47% of patients. In many cases surgery is not preferable due to risks associated with cardiac failure, further spread of infection leading to persistent sepsis due to surgical removal of an infected thrombus and/or life threatening embolisation.

Significant advances have been made recently in our understanding of the molecular mechanisms leading to disease progression thus the primary intent in producing this book is to elevate awareness and enthusiasm in the field. It is based on these recent advances that I hope it will provide greater understanding of the challenges this complex disease brings.

Dr. Steven W. Kerrigan
Principal Investigator,
Cardiovascular Infection Group,
Royal College of Surgeons in Ireland,
Dublin, Ireland

Chapter 1

Complications of Endocarditis

Yongping Wang and Aifeng Wang

Additional information is available at the end of the chapter

http://dx.doi.org/10.5772/56091

1. Introduction

Infective endocarditis (IE) is an endovascular infection and inflammation with vegetation formation, usually caused by infectious agents. Bacterial infection is most common for IE, but other pathogens such as fungi, richettsia, chlamydia and virus, can also cause IE [1]. The vegetations vary in size and shape and are composed of platelet and fibrin blocks with plenty of microbial and small amounts of inflammatory cells inside [2]. IE occurs mostly in the patients with cardiac abnormalities or lesions including rheumatic heart disease, ventricular septal defect, patent ductus arteriosus, valvular stenosis or incompetence [3]. Nevertheless, IE can also be seen in other conditions, such as valve replacement, pacemaker implantation, intravenous drug users and a few people without cardiac lesions. Most patients are young and clinically exhibit low to mild fever, progressive anemia, asthenia, night sweat, hepatosplenomegaly and clubbed finger (toe) [1-3].

The incidence of IE is 30 per million persons per year [4]. Despite major improvements in diagnosis and treatment, the mortality of IE still remains high at 14% of in-hospital and even higher at 20% to 30% complicated with age and heart failure, especially in developing countries [5,6]. Based on different criteria, IE can be divided by several classifications. By duration, IE can be classified to subacute bacterial endocarditis (SBE) and acute bacterial endocarditis (ABE); By culture result, IE can be divided by *staphylococcal* endocarditis, *streptococcal* endocarditis, *enterococcal* endocarditis, *fungal* endocarditis; By individual valve type, IE can be classified by native valve endocarditis, prosthetic valve endocarditis and endocarditis in intravenous drug abusers [2-4]. As reported in a study with an IE population of 223 episodes, complications occurred in 74% patients, including cardiac, neurological, septic, renal, embolism and infarction/ abscess [7]. It also suggests that neurologic and septic complications are the leading causes of death in IE patients [7]. With the improvement of diagnosis and therapy, the frequencies of IE complications have changed. For example, septic and embolic symptoms are relatively rare because of early and adequate dosage of antibiotic therapy [4]. On the contrary, there are increasing complications in prosthetic valve IE and intravenous drug abuse patients which may bring new challenge for clinical diagnosis and therapy. Since there are different diagnostic criteria for IE, it is difficult to conclude the true incidence of IE [8]. Overall, diagnosis is missed until autopsy in 38.2% of cases, especially when the patients are absence of fever, cardiac murmurs and other typical symptoms of IE [9]. In this chapter, several most common complications and related pathophysiologic process in IE patients will be summarized.

2. Intracardiac infection and local spread

Cardiac complications are the most common complications seen in IE patients, occurring in one-third to one-half of patients in most recent case series [10, 11].

2.1. Congestive Heart Failure (CHF)

CHF is a leading cause of death in IE patients [12]. The size of nodular or polypoid-like vegetation varies from 1 micrometer to several centimeters which can block the valve entrance [13]. The vegetation can cause valvular perforation and lead to prolapse. When the infection is controlled, valve lesions may still go on with fibrosis and contracture in some cases. All of these pathologic changes induce valvular insufficiency, mainly involved in aortic valve (50%), mitral valve (40%) and tricuspid valve (6%) [14]. A study on 511 IE patients show that moderate or severe congestive heart failure accounts for 44% in total complications [15]. According the report enrolling 4166 IE patients from multi centers in 28 countries, 33.4% patients have heart failure and 66.7% of the heart failure patients are classified as New York Heart Association class III or IV symptom status [16]. The total in-hospital mortality is 29.7% for the CHF cohort. They conclude that the severities of CHF in IE patients are associated with surgical status and mortality [16]. Based on the seriousness of CHF in the course of IE patients, the timing for early prophylaxis and treatment will influence its prognostic significance.

2.2. Cardiac abscess

Abscess is most common in acute patients and may happen anywhere in the heart [17]. The most frequent cardiac abscess occurs in aortic root of 56.5% of (26/46) IE patients, and the infecting organism is staphylococcus (52.3%) in patients with abscesses more often than in those without abscesses (16.2%) [17]. Occasionally, cardiac abscess can cause papillary muscle rupture, ventricular septal perforation, and even purulent pericarditis when the infection infiltrates the myocardial wall [13]. Moreover, the infection beyond the valve annulus can spread to adjacent structures and cause an emergency and higher mortality which can be observed in 88% of cases [18]. Another study on a large number of cases with valvular ring abscesses suggests that early identification of abscesses is particularly important to improve the outcome after timely surgery [19]. They also conclude that the overall operative mortality is not correlated with patient's age, *staphylococcal* infection or abscess fistulization [19]. However, the diagnosis is difficult, especially for small abscesses located on the anterior aortic wall and mitral abscesses.

3. Embolic

Embolization is frequently observed in IE patients and can even occur in patients undergoing therapies. IE patients have high prevalence of embolic complications for 13-49% [20]. In a study of 65 IE patients, a total of 37 (56.9%) patients are diagnosed with a cerebral embolism (overt 13, clinically silent 24) by blood test, cultures, echocardiography, and MRI/CT imaging [21]. Their results suggest that both overt and clinical silent central nervous system embolism are common complications of IE patients and silent embolism needs further imaging tools for examination [21]. Recently, their group uses some new biological markers, such as S-100B, to predict embolism in central nervous system during the course of IE [22]. Since most of the S-100B protein are synthesized by astrocytes and released from damaged neural tissues, the biomarker provides another specific method for screening CNS stroke in IE patients. An early study shows that the microorganism, but not vegetations on echocardiography, is associated with a significantly higher risk for embolus in patients with left-sided IE [23]. With transthoracic echocardiography in predicting embolic events, another group found that the vegetations bigger than 10 mm were associated with a 50% incidence of embolic events, while vegetations less than 10 mm had a 42% incidence of emboli in IE patients [24]. Similarly, in the patients who are diagnosed with acute IE and have no confirmed or suspected embolism before, 44% (25 in 57) have embolic events by using both transthoracic and transesophageal echocardiograms [25]. They also suggest the characteristics of vegetations identified by echocardiograms are not helpful in predicting embolic risk in IE patients [25]. In combination with clinical antibiotic therapy, embolism occurred in 34.1% (131 in 384) patients before/after IE diagnosis and in 7.3% (28 in 384) patients after initiation of therapy [26].

Besides neurological embolism, other organs such as spleen, kidney, lung and limbs, are also involved in rare cases [27, 28]. According to a report by Luaces-Méndez *et al*, there are 10% hepatosplenic and renal embolisms infarctions in left-sided IE patients with characteristic clinical features [29]. But in fungi caused IE, emboli occurs in 25%(41 in 162) patients and symptomatic embolization appears to be more common of 17% (7 in 41) in peripheral limb, 7% (3 in 41) in pulmonary, 5% (2 in 41) in mesenteric [30].

The characteristics of bacterial embolus are multiple, fragile and movable, so in many cases IE patients present with stroke, meningitis, brain abscess and bacterial aneurysm.

3.1. Stroke

Ischemic and hemorrhagic strokes are important neurological complications and are frequent in IE patients during uncontrolled infection. There are about 21% complicated by stroke in 212 IE patients in a study between 1978 and 1986 [31]. In a population of 214 IE patients undergoing cardiac surgery, the prognosis for patients with uncomplicated ischemic stroke are better than patients with complicated stroke (meningitis, hemorrhage, or brain abscess) after 20 years following up [32]. In order to prevent cardioembolic stroke, additional diagnostic tools such as echocardiography and cardiac magnetic resonance imaging, can be applied to identify the sources of cardiac embolism. Another investigation in 707 patients who are diagnosed with possible IE, strokes occur in 9.6% of total cases, which is lower than previous reports (21 to 39%) [33]. In order to study the relationship between vegetation 2-dimensional size and stroke in those IE patients, researchers use Duke Endocarditis Database to examine 145 IE patients and find 23.4% (34 in 145) complicated by stroke, suggesting vegetation 2-dimensional size and characteristics as predictors for stroke and mortality [34].

3.2. Mycotic aneurysm

If the artery is blocked by the septic embolus, the wall may be necrosised and destroyed, and then develop bacterial aneurysm. Mycotic aneurysm is rare, about 4% (23 in 513), in IE patients [15]. Aorta, brain, viscera and limbs can become involved in turn [35]. Patients can show throbbing lump during the late stage. The disease is easily diagnosed while occuring at peripheral vessels. However, when the lesion happens in deep arteries such as brain and mesentery, aneurysm is always ignored until it is broken and bleeding [36]. Mycotic aneurysm has a high mortality rate for its potential catastrophic rupture but can be prevented by early diagnostic imaging techniques [37]. Cerebral mycotic aneurysms tend to occur in the more distal portions of the middle cerebral artery, especially in the region of the sylvian fissure, which clinically is different from berry aneurysms occurring near the Willis circle [38].

3.3. Cerebral hemorrhage

Cerebral hemorrhage will occur when the vessel is broken in bacterial aneurysm or embolism. It is easy to develop spotted or patched hemorrhage when there is big area of infarction in the brain. There are three different mechanisms for cerebral haemorrhage in IE patients: rupture of a mycotic aneurysm, septic arteritis without aneurysm, spontaneous haemorrhagic transformation of a blank brain infarction [39].

Subarachnoid hemorrhage is a rare but dramatic neurologic complication in IE patients and is always associated with aneurysm rupture in the early phase [40]. Previous reports show that high mortality is related to intracerebral haemorrhage [41, 42]. The species of microorganism seem to have relationship with brain haemorrhage. Data presented in an investigation shows that brain haemorrhages in 40.7% (35 in 86) IE patients are caused by *Staphylococcus aures* [43].

4. Hematogenous dissemination

4.1. Metastatic abscess

When the vegetation with infecting bacteria drops off, it will migrate with blood and cause embolism in the artery. During a report on 118 IE patients, 44 (37.3 %) patients have 46 definite regions of abscess in total and abscesses present more frequently in endocarditis from aortic-valve than other valves [17]. If the infection is not controlled well, abscesses can develop in the spleen, kidney, brain or soft tissues in IE patients. With the improvement of antibiotic treatment, metastatic abscess is relatively rare but still reported in recent years [44-46].

Splenic abscesses are found in up to 5% IE patients and usually exhibit abdominal pain, pleuritic or shoulder pain as of diaphragmatic irritation, or persistent fever [47]. According to the conclusion from 27 patients with splenic abscess, the cases could not survive without a timely splenectomy surgery [48]. If possible, the patient with IE should be treated first for splenic abscesses and then splenectomy should be performed for the requirements.[49].

Cerebral abscess is rare in IE patients including suppurative encephalitis, chronic granuloma and abscess envelope [50]. The time for envelope formation depends on the types of bacteria and the toxicity, body's resistance and reaction for antibiotic therapy [51]. According to the report on a series of cases, miliary microscopic abscesses are more common than macroscopic cerebral abscess in bacterial endocarditis patients, particularly in patients with acute miliary infection [41]. Cerebral abscesses in some IE patients are suggested to be related with *S. aureus* infection and purulent meningitis [41].

4.2. Toxic encephalopathy

Toxic encephalopathy occurs when plenty of bacteria enter the circulation and cause septicemia. In an investigation of 110 patients, 19.1% (21 in 110) show toxic encephalopathy, which is ranked the second common neurological manifestation of IE patients [52]. Frequently, the patients display a variety of symptoms, such as early stage of headache, dizziness, hypersomnia, nausea, vomit and late stage of hallucination, memory loss, small personality changes, seizures, disturbance of consciousness. The multiple cerebral emboli and multifocal microinfarcts cause formation of microabscesses, which may explain the pathophysiological mechanism for acute encephalopathy [53].

4.3. Purulent meningitis

This complication is uncommon and concomitant with cerebral abscess. Sometimes the intracerebral abscess may enter subarachnoid cavity and cerebral ventricle to invade meninges, which will cause purulent meningitis [54]. If *Streptococcus anaerobius, bacteroid, Staphylococcus* and mixed bacteria are separated in cerebrospinal fluid, it suggests that there are relationships between meningitis and broken intracerebral abscess.

5. Musculoskeletal complications

The musculoskeletal manifestations include spondylodiscitis, osteomyelitis, septic arthritis and peripheral soft tissue abscess, which occur frequently in up to 44% cases [55]. Because the existing of osteoarticular complications, the patients are at a higher risk of having major embolic events from the central nerve system to lungs [56]. Vertebral osteomyelitis is relatively rare complication in IE patients. Overall, 4.6% (28 in 606) cases in IE patients have pyegenic vertebral osteomyelitis [57]. The patients are needed to exclude IE if they have spondylodiscitis and pre-existing heart disease or microbiologic infection [58]. With MRI as a highly sensitive and specific tool for diagnosing, patients with spondylodiscitis usually can be found early before infection has spread to two vertebral body levels.

In IE patients, the percentages of osteomyelitis and septic arthritis are up to 4.3%, and they occur more frequently in patients with tricuspid valve involvement [56]. *S. aureus* are reported to have higher frequencies than other microorganisms for causing osteomyelitis complication in IE patients [59]. The infections usually occur at large joints and involve one or more joints, including the knee, shoulder, elbow, hip and sacroiliac joints [56]. If the patients are infected with multiple joints but don't have joint infection or trauma, they are suspicious for septic arthritis with IE.

6. Immune-mediated damage

With persistent bacteremia existing in IE patients, clinical manifestations, such as splenomegaly, glomerulonephritis and arthritis, may present because of cellular and humoral-mediated immune response [60]. Patients with splenomegaly occur in 20% of cases and are more likely in patients who have been ill for months rather than for days or weeks. Glomerulonephritis are most common in *S. aureus* caused ABE and *S. viridans* caused SBE with histologic immune deposits in the glomerular capillary wall [61]. With antibiotic prophylaxis and therapy in IE patients, the incidence of glomerulonephritis decreases to about 4.5% (9 in 198) in an investigation [62]. Under rare conditions, patients with glomerulonephritis will develop diffuse proliferative glomerulonephritis and extensive crescent formation with renal failure [63].

Other clinical manifestations, such as arthritis, pericarditis and micro-vessel vasculitis are also found in IE patients. Vasculitis may cause unspecific signs on skin and mucosa, including subconjunctival and soft palate petechiae, hemorrhages within the nail beds (splinter hemorrhages), oval retinal bleeding spots with white center (Roth spots), painful subcutaneous nodules on the palms or soles (Osler's nodes), painless bleeding spots on the palms and soles with diameter of 1 to 4 mm (Janeway lesions) [1]. The pathogenesis for above lesions may be caused by microemboli and microabscesses in the small vessels of dermis.

In summary, multidisciplinary approaches including clinician microbiologists, radiology, cardiology and surgery are necessary for treatment of IE with complications. In order to get better understanding, the complications are classified into several categories although some features are overlapping or broad. For example, the IE patients with embolic complication can have metastatic abscess, mycotic aneurysm or cerebral hemorrhage; patients with hematogenous dissemination can simultaneously have embolic and musculoskeletal symptoms. This content tries to describe the frequency of IE complications and may help for better prophylaxis and therapy.

Acknowledgements

We are grateful to Zhijian Duan at UC Davis for reviewing and editing this chapter. Yongping Wang is supported by grant from the Shriners Hospital for Children [84204 to Y.P.W].

Author details

Yongping Wang[1,2*] and Aifeng Wang[3,4]

*Address all correspondence to: wypwang@ucdavis.edu

1 Department of Cell Biology and Human Anatomy, University of California, Davis, USA

2 Institute of Pediatric Regenerative Medicine, Shriners Hospital for Children-North California, University of California, Davis, USA

3 Department of Biochemistry and Molecular Medicine, University of California, Davis, USA

4 Department of Forensic Medicine, Preclinical Medical College, Southern Medical University, Guangzhou, Guangdong, China

References

[1] Baddour LM, Wilson WR, Bayer AS, Fowler VG Jr, Bolger AF, Levison ME, et al. Council on Cardiovascular Disease in the Young; Councils on Clinical Cardiology, Stroke, and Cardiovascular Surgery and Anesthesia; American Heart Association; Infectious Diseases Society of America. Infective endocarditis: diagnosis, antimicrobial therapy, and management of complications: a statement for healthcare professionals from the Committee on Rheumatic Fever, Endocarditis, and Kawasaki Disease, Council on Cardiovascular Disease in the Young, and the Councils on Clinical Cardiology, Stroke, and Cardiovascular Surgery and Anesthesia, American Heart Association: endorsed by the Infectious Diseases Society of America. *Circulation* 2005, 111: e394-434.

[2] Bayer AS, Bolger AF, Taubert KA, Wilson W, Steckelberg J, Karchmer AW, et al. Diagnosis and management of infective endocarditis and its complications. *Circulation* 1998, 98: 2936-2948.

[3] Horstkotte D, Follath F, Gutschik E, Lengyel M, Oto A, Pavie A, et al. Guidelines on prevention, diagnosis and treatment of infective endocarditis: executive summary; the Task Force on Infective Endocarditis of the European Society of Cardiology. *Eur Heart J* 2004, 25: 267-276.

[4] Mylonakis E, Calderwood SB. Infective endocarditis in adults. *N Engl J Med* 2001, 345: 1318-1330.

[5] Tariq M, Alam M, Munir G, Khan MA, Smego RA Jr. Infective endocarditis: a five-year experience at a tertiary care hospital in Pakistan. *Int J Infect Dis* 2004, 8: 163-170.

[6] Fedeli U, Schievano E, Buonfrate D, Pellizzer G, Spolaore P. Increasing incidence and mortality of infective endocarditis: a population-based study through a record-linkage system. *BMC Infect Dis* 2011, 11: 48.

[7] Mansur AJ, Grinberg M, da Luz PL, Bellotti G. The complications of infective endocarditis. A reappraisal in the 1980s. *Arch Intern Med* 1992, 152: 2428-2432.

[8] Heiro M, Nikoskelainen J, Hartiala JJ, Saraste MK, Kotilainen PM. Diagnosis of infective endocarditis. Sensitivity of the Duke vs von Reyn criteria. *Arch Intern Med* 1998, 158: 18-24.

[9] Fernández Guerrero ML, Álvarez B, Manzarbeitia F, Renedo G. Infective endocarditis at autopsy: a review of pathologic manifestations and clinical correlates. *Medicine (Baltimore)* 2012, 91: 152-164.

[10] Millaire A, Van Belle E, de Groote P, Leroy O, Ducloux G. Obstruction of the left main coronary ostium due to an aortic vegetation: survival after early surgery. *Clin Infect Dis* 1996, 22: 192-193.

[11] Nadji G, Rusinaru D, Rémadi JP, Jeu A, Sorel C, Tribouilloy C. Heart failure in left-sided native valve infective endocarditis: characteristics, prognosis, and results of surgical treatment. *Eur J Heart Fail* 2009, 11: 668-675.

[12] Delahaye F, Alla F, Béguinot I, Bruneval P, Doco-Lecompte T, Lacassin F, et al. In-hospital mortality of infective endocarditis: prognostic factors and evolution over an 8-year period. *Scand J Infect Dis* 2007, 39: 849-857.

[13] Bashore TM, Cabell C, Fowler V Jr. Update on infective endocarditis. *Curr Probl Cardiol* 2006, 31: 274-352.

[14] Lalani T, Cabell CH, Benjamin DK, Lasca O, Naber C, Fowler VG Jr, et al. International Collaboration on Endocarditis-Prospective Cohort Study (ICE-PCS) Investigators. Analysis of the impact of early surgery on in-hospital mortality of native valve endocarditis: use of propensity score and instrumental variable methods to adjust for treatment-selection bias. *Circulation* 2010, 121: 1005-1013.

[15] Hasbun R, Vikram HR, Barakat LA, Buenconsejo J, Quagliarello VJ. Complicated left-sided native valve endocarditis in adults: risk classification for mortality. *JAMA* 2003, 289: 1933-1940.

[16] Kiefer T, Park L, Tribouilloy C, Cortes C, Casillo R, Chu V, et al. Association between valvular surgery and mortality among patients with infective endocarditis complicated by heart failure. *JAMA* 2011, 306: 2239-2247.

[17] Daniel WG, Mugge A, Martin RP, Lindert O, Hausmann D, Nonnast-Daniel B, et al. Improvement in the diagnosis of abscesses associated with endocarditis by transesophageal echocardiography. *N Engl J Med* 1991, 324: 795-800.

[18] Sampedro MF, Patel R. Infections associated with long-term prosthetic devices. *Infect Dis Clin North Am* 2007, 21: 785-819.

[19] Choussat R, Thomas D, Isnard R, Michel PL, Iung B, Hanania G, et al. Perivalvular abscesses associated with endocarditis; clinical features and prognostic factors of overall survival in a series of 233 cases. Perivalvular Abscesses French Multicentre Study. *Eur Heart J* 1999, 20: 232-241.

[20] Habib G. Embolic risk of subacute bacterial endocarditis: role of transesophageal echocardiography. *Curr Cardiol Rep* 2003, 5: 129-136.

[21] Grabowski M, Hryniewiecki T, Janas J, Stępińska J. Clinically overt and silent cerebral embolism in the course of infective endocarditis. *J Neurol* 2011, 258: 1133-1139.

[22] Grabowski M, Hryniewiecki T, Stępińska J. Novel markers of cerebral embolism in the course of infective endocarditis. *Int J Cardiol* 2012, 154: 90-92.

[23] Steckelberg JM, Murphy JG, Ballard D, Bailey K, Tajik AJ, Taliercio CP, et al. Emboli in infective endocarditis: the prognostic value of echocardiography. *Ann Intern Med* 1991, 114: 635-640.

[24] Heinle S, Wilderman N, Harrison JK, Waugh R, Bashore T, Nicely LM, et al. Value of transthoracic echocardiography in predicting embolic events in active infective endocarditis. Duke Endocarditis Service. *Am J Cardiol* 1994, 74: 799-801.

[25] De Castro S, Magni G, Beni S, Cartoni D, Fiorelli M, Venditti M, et al. Role of transthoracic and transesophageal echocardiography in predicting embolic events in patients with active infective endocarditis involving native cardiac valves. Am J Cardiol 1997, 80: 1030-1034.

[26] Thuny F, Di Salvo G, Belliard O, Avierinos JF, Pergola V, Rosenberg V, et al. Risk of embolism and death in infective endocarditis: prognostic value of echocardiography: a prospective multicenter study. *Circulation* 2005, 112: 69-75.

[27] Pessinaba S, Kane A, Ndiaye MB, Mbaye A, Bodian M, Dia MM, et al. Vascular complications of infective endocarditis. *Med Mal Infect* 2012, 42: 213-217.

[28] Ting W, Silverman NA, Arzouman DA, Levitsky S. Splenic septic emboli in endocarditis. *Circulation* 1990, 82: IV105-109.

[29] Luaces Méndez M, Vilacosta I, Sarriá C, Fernández C, San Román JA, Sanmartín JV, et al. Hepatosplenic and renal embolisms in infective endocarditis. *Rev Esp Cardiol* 2004, 57: 1188-1196.

[30] Ellis ME, Al-Abdely H, Sandridge A, Greer W, Ventura W. Fungal endocarditis: evidence in the world literature, 1965-1995. *Clin Infect Dis* 2001, 32: 50-62.

[31] Hart RG, Foster JW, Luther MF, Kanter MC. Stroke in infective endocarditis. *Stroke* 1990, 21: 695-700.

[32] Ruttmann E, Willeit J, Ulmer H, Chevtchik O, Höfer D, Poewe W, et al. Neurological outcome of septic cardioembolic stroke after infective endocarditis. *Stroke* 2006, 37: 2094-2099.

[33] Anderson DJ, Goldstein LB, Wilkinson WE, Corey GR, Cabell CH, Sanders LL, et al. Stroke location, characterization, severity, and outcome in mitral vs. aortic valve endocarditis. *Neurology* 2003, 61:1341-1346.

[34] Cabell CH, Pond KK, Peterson GE, Durack DT, Corey GR, Anderson DJ, et al. The risk of stroke and death in patients with aortic and mitral valve endocarditis. *Am Heart J* 2001, 142: 75-80.

[35] Dubois M, Daenens K, Houthoofd S, Peetermans WE, Fourneau I. Treatment of mycotic aneurysms with involvement of the abdominal aorta: single-centre experience in 44 consecutive cases. *Eur J Vasc Endovasc Surg* 2010, 40: 450-456.

[36] Ziment, I. Nervous system complications in bacterial endocarditis. Am J Med 1969; 47:593.

[37] Shaikholeslami R, Tomlinson CW, Teoh KH, Molot MJ, Duke RJ. Mycotic aneurysm complicating staphylococcal endocarditis. *Can J Cardiol* 1999, 15: 217-222.

[38] Jones HR Jr, Siekert RG. Neurological manifestations of infective endocarditis: Review of clinical and therapeutic challenges. *Brain* 1989, 112: 1295-1315.

[39] Hart RG, Kagan-Hallet K, Joerns SE. Mechanisms of intracranial hemorrhage in infective endocarditis. *Stroke* 1987, 18: 1048-1056.

[40] Kanter MC, Hart RG. Neurologic complications of infective endocarditis. *Neurology* 1991, 41: 1015-1020.

[41] Pruitt AA, Rubin RH, Karchmer AW, Duncan GW. Neurologic complications of bacterial endocarditis. *Medicine (Baltimore)* 1978, 57:329-343.

[42] Heiro M, Nikoskelainen J, Engblom E, Kotilainen E, Marttila R, Kotilainen P. Neurologic manifestations of infective endocarditis: a 17-year experience in a teaching hospital in Finland. *Arch Intern Med* 2000, 160: 2781-2787.

[43] LeCam B, Guivarch G, Boles JM, Garre M, Cartier F. Neurologic complications in a group of 86 bacterial endocarditis. *Eur Heart J* 1984, 5 (Suppl C): 97-100.

[44] Wang CC, Lee CH, Chan CY, Chen HW. Splenic infarction and abscess complicating infective endocarditis. *Am J Emerg Med* 2009, 27: 1021.e3-5.

[45] Wadhwa R, Thakur JD, Nanda A, Guthikonda B. Sterile hemorrhagic brain abscess in infective endocarditis. *Neurol India* 2012, 60: 240-242.

[46] Kanter MC, Hart RG. Neurologic complications of infective endocarditis. *Neurology*, 1991, 41: 1015–1020.

[47] Mansur AJ, Grinberg M, da Luz PL, Bellotti G. The complications of infective endocarditis. A reappraisal in the 1980s. *Arch Intern Med* 1992, 152: 2428–2432.

[48] Robinson, SL, Saxe, JM, Lucus, CE, Arbulu A, Ledgerwood AM, Lucas WF. Splenic abscess associated with endocarditis. *Surgery* 1992, 112: 781-786.

[49] Bayer AS, Bolger AF, Taubert KA, Wilson W, Steckelberg J, Karchmer AW, et al. Diagnosis and management of infective endocarditis and its complications. *Circulation* 1998, 98: 2936-2948.

[50] Muzumdar D, Jhawar S, Goel A. Brain abscess: an overview. *Int J Surg* 2011, 9: 136-144. Epub 2010 Nov 16.

[51] Mathisen GE, Johnson JP. Brain abscess. *Clin Infect Dis* 1997, 25: 763-779.

[52] Jones HR Jr, Siekert RG, Geraci JE. Neurologic manifestations of bacterial endocarditis. *Annals of Internal Medicine* 1969, 71: 21-28.

[53] Jones HR Jr, Siekert RG. Neurological manifestations of infective endocarditis. Review of clinical and therapeutic challenges. *Brain* 1989, 112: 1295-1315.

[54] Heiro M, Nikoskelainen J, Engblom E, Kotilainen E, Marttila R, Kotilainen P. Neurologic manifestations of infective endocarditis. *Arch Intern Med* 2000, 160: 2781–2787.

[55] Churchill MA Jr, Geraci JE, Hunder GG. Musculoskeletal manifestations of bacterial endocarditis. *Ann Intern Med* 1977, 87: 754–759.

[56] Lamas C, Boia M, Eykyn SJ. Osteoarticular infections complicating infective endocarditis: a study of 30 cases between 1969 and 2002 in a tertiary referral centre. *Scand J Infect Dis* 2006, 38: 433–440.

[57] Pigrau C, Almirante B, Flores X, Falco V, Rodripuez D, Gasser I, et al. Spontaneous pyogenic vertebral osteomyelitis and endocarditis: incidence, risk factors, and outcome. *Am J Med* 2005, 118:1287.

[58] Morelli S, Carmenini E, Caporossi AP, Aguglia G, Bernardo ML, Gurgo AM. Spondylodiscitis and infective endocarditis: case studies and review of the literature. *Spine* 2001, 26: 499–500.

[59] Di Salvo G, Habib G, Pergola V, Avierinos JF, Philip E, Casalta JP. Echocardiography predicts embolic events in infective endocarditis. *J Am Coll Cardiol* 2001, 37: 1069-1076.

[60] Burton-Kee J, Morgan-Capner P, Mowbray JF. Nature of circulating immune complexes in infective endocarditis. *J Clin Pathol* 1980, 33: 653-659.

[61] Neugarten J, Baldwin DS. Glomerulonephritis in bacterial endocarditis. *Am J Med.* 1984, 77: 297-304.

[62] Garg N, Kandpal B, Garg N, Tewari S, Kapoor A, Goel P, et al. Characteristics of infective endocarditis in a developing country-clinical profile and outcome in 192 Indian patients, 1992-2001. *Int J Cardiol* 2005, 98: 253-260.

[63] Kannan S, Mattoo TK. Diffuse crescentic glomerulonephritis in bacterial endocarditis. *Pediatr Nephrol* 2001, 16: 423-428.

Chapter 2

Platelet-Bacterial Interactions in the Pathogenesis of Infective Endocarditis — Part I: The Streptococcus

Dorothea Tilley and Steven W. Kerrigan

Additional information is available at the end of the chapter

http://dx.doi.org/10.5772/55912

1. Introduction

Infective endocarditis (IE) is a life threatening disease caused by a bacterial infection of the endocardial surfaces of the heart. It is typified by the formation of septic thrombi or vegetative growth on the heart valve. Typically, both platelets and fibrin are deposited on exposed extracellular matrix proteins as part of the normal response to damage of the endocardium [1]. However, this sterile platelet-fibrin nidus facilitates colonisation of the endocardium by bacteria in the bloodstream [2]. Following attachment, bacteria can recruit platelets from the circulation inducing platelet activation and platelet aggregation. This results in the development of large macroscopic vegetations which resist infiltration by both immune cells and antibiotics making IE a difficult disease to treat. These vegetations commonly occur on the heart valves and can disrupt hemodynamic patterns within the heart. This puts undue force on often already compromised valves, leading to congestive heart failure [3]. IE is notoriously difficult to treat, requiring aggressive multi-antibiotic therapy often coupled with surgery to remove vegetations and/or replace the infected valve [4]. Therapy is successful when all traces of bacteria are absent from the blood stream. Multiple species of bacteria have been isolated from the infected vegetations of patients [5, 6] with IE but the streptococci are amongst the most common cause, second only to the staphylococci whose interactions with human platelets are discussed elsewhere in this book (Chapter X). Indeed, in a recent prospective study, the role of streptococci in IE is masked by the growing incidence of staphylococcal IE resulting from the increased use of medical procedures leaving streptococci as a main cause of IE in the normal population [7, 8].

2. The Streptococcus

The streptococci are a large family of gram positive coccus shaped bacteria that reside in the mouth, intestine, upper respiratory tract and the skin. Most have a commensal relationship with their host. However, as opportunistic pathogens they can cause disease if they gain access to normally sterile sites of the body such as the bloodstream. Most streptococci isolated from patients with IE are of oral origin [9], normally found colonising the salivary tooth pellicle through the interactions of surface expressed virulence factors, called adhesins, with specific moieties or motifs on host proteins or cells. When these streptococci enter the bloodstream these bacterial components participate in additional interactions with platelets. Whether this is by design or simply as a consequence of conserved motifs within the human host is unknown but regardless their interaction with human platelets is a key step in the pathogenesis of IE.

3. Platelet biology I: Haemostatic function

In the absence of infection, platelets act as sentinels of vascular integrity, patrolling the endothelium for sites of damage. Upon vascular damage these small anucleate cells interact with exposed extracellular matrix proteins via specific receptors expressed on their surface and a complex yet coordinated series of interactions and signalling events proceed, culminating in the formation of a haemostatic plug. Platelet receptor complex GPIb-IX-V recognises von Willebrand Factor (vWF) bound to exposed collagen fibrils in the subendothelial matrix, tethering the platelet to the site of damage [10, 11]. This initial interaction is relatively weak and has a fast on-off rate [12] so the platelet characteristically rolls along the endothelium breaking and remaking the vWF-GPIb-IV-X interaction [1]. This 'rolling' mechanism slows the platelet sufficiently for additional receptor-ligand contacts and triggers an intracellular signal resulting in integrin activation and firm adhesion. Firm adhesion is mediated by a combination of ligand receptor engagements: integrin $\alpha2\beta1$ - collagen [13-15]; glycoprotein GPVI - collagen [16]; $\alpha5\beta1$-fibronectin [17]; and $\alpha IIb\beta3$ with fibrinogen and vWF [12, 18]. Once firmly adhered, the platelet undergoes dramatic rearrangement of its cytoskeleton causing platelet shape change from its resting discoid form to a dendritic form and finally, to a fully spread platelet with characteristic filipodia and llamelipodia [19]. During this process, the platelet secretes signalling molecules, proteins and platelet agonists (ADP, ATP and serotonin) from its cytoplasmic granules (α- and dense- granules) and synthesizes and secretes thromboxane, amplifying the platelet response, recruiting and activating nearby platelets. Activated platelets can undergo platelet aggregation, cross linking with one another via their $\alpha IIb\beta3$ receptors and the divalent plasma protein fibrinogen. This activation and recruitment of platelets to the site of injury, in addition to stimulation of the coagulation system and formation of a fibrin network, forms the haemostatic plug.

4. Platelet biology II: Immune function

The platelet role in haemostasis and thrombosis is well characterised but, at the same time, their activities can be viewed from an immunological perspective [20]. Their primary role of maintaining vascular integrity is an essential process in preventing entry of foreign particles into the blood stream. The epithelial barrier performs a similar function. More specifically, however, they produce antimicrobial peptides [21]; possess pathogen recognition receptors (TLRs)[22, 23]; secrete immunomodulatory molecules [24]; and have specific receptors for chemokines [25], antibody complexes [26] and complement factors [27]. Critically, as outlined in this chapter, they interact with and respond to bacteria, all hallmarks of true immune cells. It is this response, or activation, that is important in the context of IE and provides the basis for the formation of platelet-bacterial vegetations which characterise this disease.

5. Platelet-bacterial interactions: General observations

Platelet interactions are examined under the broad headings of platelet adhesion, activation and aggregation. Platelet aggregometry is a useful tool in assessing platelet activation. In contrast to conventional stimuli such as ADP and thrombin, there is a significant lag time to the onset of platelet aggregation in response to bacteria [28].The length of this lag is defined by the sum of platelet-bacterial interactions occurring and can vary between donors, most likely due to variation in the levels of platelet receptors expressed on the surface and the concentration of plasma proteins. Platelet-bacterial interactions can be categorized into direct, indirect or mediated by a secreted bacterial product [29]. A direct interaction occurs when a bacterial adhesin binds directly to a platelet receptor or other surface expressed component [30]. Bacteria can participate in indirect interactions with platelets through a bridging protein which binds to the bacterium and then to its cognate platelet receptor [31]. When bacteria enter the bloodstream they can bind plasma proteins through specific plasma binding proteins or they can simply be recognised by soluble elements of the immune system such as immunoglobulins and complement proteins. Finally, and less common for the streptococcal bacteria, a secreted bacterial product may bind to the platelet causing activation independently of bacterial attachment. The ability of bacteria to propagate platelet activation and aggregation facilitates growth of the vegetation and effectively encapsulates the bacteria, hiding them from conventional immune cells and bacterial killing mechanisms. This chapter will focus on the specific molecular events that lead to initiation of IE, namely recognition of the platelet by the bacteria (and vice versa) and the ensuing intracellular signalling events that lead to platelet activation and amplification of the platelet response. As will be evident from the discussion to follow, platelet bacterial interactions are heterogeneous in nature and additionally they are multifactorial, with most bacteria interacting with platelets through more than one mechanism.

6. Streptococcus — Platelet interactions

6.1. Early findings

Streptococcus sanguinis (formally *Streptococcus sanguis*) is the most common *Streptococcus* isolated from the valves of patients with IE [9]. Early studies identified a 115 kDa cell membrane protein that induced platelet aggregation in platelet rich plasma [32]. This rhamnose rich, platelet-aggregation associated protein (PAAP) is glycosylated and was amongst the first identified bacterial glycoproteins [33]. Bacterial glycoproteins are now thought to be almost ubiquitous, performing critical roles in host adhesion, resistance to complement killing, maintenance of cell shape and enzymatic activities that release nutrients from complex carbohydrates [34]. The platelet receptor for this protein has not been confirmed, however, an early study showed that *S. sanguinis* did not induce platelet aggregation in a patient who failed to respond to collagen suggesting the role of a collagen receptor, possibly $\alpha_2\beta_1$ [35]. Additionally, Gong et al. isolated platelet membrane proteins of molecular weights 175 kDa, 150 kDa and 230 kDa that interacted with *S. sanguinis* 133-79 [36]. The platelet binding domain of PAAP has been isolated to a 23 kDa fragment [37]. Furthermore, the peptide sequence PGEQGPK within this fragment conforms to the platelet interactive domain of collagen types I and III, KPGEPGPK, and antibodies directed against this peptide delayed the onset of aggregation induced by *S. sanguinis* [38, 39]. More recently, in an effort to identify the PAAP gene, a putative collagen binding protein was identified containing two PAAP-like sequences and platelet aggregation in platelet rich plasma was significantly reduced in response to a mutant lacking this protein while no changes in platelet adhesion were observed [40]. In conjunction with the study of Gong et al., this confirmed that *S. sanguinis* had at least one other adhesin for human platelets.

6.2. Serine rich repeat glycoproteins

The serine rich repeat (SRR) proteins are a large family of glycosylated bacterial adhesins. SRR proteins of *S. sanguinis* and its close relative *S. gordonii* mediate direct binding of these bacteria to platelets through sialic acid residues on the GPIbα subunit of the GPIb-V-IX complex [41-43].

Fimbriae-associated protein 1 (Fap1) of *S. parasanguinis* FW213 was the first SRR protein to be identified and, while it is reported not to interact with human platelets, studies of Fap1 have provided important information on the structure of SRR proteins and the nature of their ligand interactions. SRR proteins share a common domain structure: an N-terminal signal sequence; a short serine rich repeat region (SR1); a non-repetitive ligand binding region (BR); a larger serine rich repeat domain (SR2); and a cell wall anchor domain (CW) [41-47]. Like PAAP, SRR proteins are highly glycosylated. The serine rich repeat domains are decorated with O-linked carbohydrate residues [48] and the larger SR2 domain is thought to form a stalk like structure, extending the adhesive N-terminal region from the cell surface. Fap1 is critical for *S. parasanguinis* adhesion to saliva coated hydroxyapatite (sHA) and biofilm formation [49, 50]. However, Fap1 mediated adhesion to sHA is independent of these glycosylations as shown by mutation of upstream glycosyltransferases critical for glycosylation of the native protein and subsequent biofilm formation [51].

In contrast to the conserved structural organisation of SRR proteins, the peptide sequence of the non repetitive region varies significantly and is suggested to explain the differing affinity of SRR proteins to platelets and other cell types. To date only the SRR proteins of *S. sanguinis* (SrpA) and *S. gordonii* (GspB and Hsa) have been demonstrated to interact directly with human platelets while others, PsrP of *S. pneumoniae* and Srr-1 of *S. agalactiae* bind to keratin 10 and 4 in lung epithelial and endothelial cells respectively [52, 53]. The platelet interactive domains and specifically the sialic acid binding domain of GspB and Hsa are isolated to the non repetitive region [43]. Most recently, x-ray crystallography studies of the non-repetitive ligand binding region of GspB have revealed a modular organization: helical domain; a domain similar to the binding domain of *Staphylococcus aureus* collagen binding protein CnaA; a Siglec domain; and a Unique domain [54]. Interestingly, the Siglec domain, a mammalian carbohydrate binding domain, was found in Hsa and SrpA but not in the protein sequences of five other characterised SRR proteins suggesting that this domain is critical for interactions with GPIbα [54]. Indeed, a point mutation (R484E) in the Siglec domain showed a marked reduction in binding to glycocalicin, the ectodomain of GPIbα and reduced bacterial load in the vegetations of a catheterized rat model of infective endocarditis [54].

GPIbα is a glycosylated, type one transmembrane receptor. A long highly glycosylated region called the macroglobulin region, or mucin-like core, extends from the cell surface presenting ligand binding domains to the extracellular milieu [55]. The macroglobulin region is decorated in predominantly O-linked but some N-linked carbohydrates terminating in sialic acid[55]. This highly glycosylated protein backbone is followed by a sulphated tyrosine region, a leucine rich repeat domain and an N-terminal domain decorated with N-linked sialic acid oligosaccharides [55]. Hsa is proposed to bind to both the N-terminal domain and the macroglobulin region while GspB interactions are isolated to the macroglobulin stalk [43]. Further complexity is added as GspB and Hsa display distinct preferences for O-linked and N-linked glycosylations respectively [43]. The subtle differences in binding affinity of SrpA to sialic acid moieties remain to be elucidated but studies using anti-GPIbα site specific antibodies isolated the *S. sanguinis* interactive region of GPIbα to the N-terminal region and the sulphated tyrosine region [30]. This suggests that SrpA interacts with human platelets in a distinct mechanism to GspB and Hsa. However, the ability to bind sialic acid residues is critical as sialidase treated platelets and glycocalicin support significantly less bacterial binding than the untreated samples [41-43]. In platelet function studies, deletion of either Hsa or SrpA failed to prevent platelet aggregation suggesting other platelet-bacterial interactions are needed to induce platelet activation [41, 56]. In contrast, using an *in vitro* model of blood flow, platelets were observed rolling before stably adhering to *S. sanguinis* 133-79 [41]. This is characteristic of GPIbα interactions with vWF under shear conditions. When platelets were perfused over an immobilised strain of *S. sanguinis* defective in expression of SrpA or an *S. gordonii* strain defective in Hsa expression, no rolling or attachment was observed suggesting that these SRR are essential for initial platelet attachment in the blood stream [41, 56].

7. Antigen I/II family of bacterial adhesins

The antigen I/II family of proteins are ubiquitous to streptococci being found in most published genomes to date with roles in the development of microbial communities and adhesion to host cells and proteins [57]. Like the SRR proteins they share a common domain organisation: a signal sequence; an N-terminal region; an alanine rich repeat domain; a variable domain; a proline rich repeat region; a C-terminal region and a cell wall anchor domain [58].

Investigation of the role of the antigen I/II family of adhesins in *S. gordonii*-platelet interactions was prompted by the observation that, while adhesion to *S. gordonii* DL1 was reduced by mutation of Hsa, the platelet aggregation response remained, suggesting a second interaction [56]. Indeed, a proteomic approach using cell wall extracts from an aggregating *S. gordonii* strain (DL1) and a non aggregating strain (Blackburn) revealed two antigen I/II proteins of molecular weights 172 kDa and 164 kDa [56]. These were designated SspA and SspB [56]. Mutation of these proteins did not affect platelet adhesion to wildtype *S. gordonii* or, indeed, a Hsa mutant. However, platelet aggregation was completely abolished when Hsa, SspA and SspB were mutated simultaneously [56, 59]. SspA and SspB participate in fluid phase interactions with salivary glycoprotein gp340, facilitating bacterial clumping which most likely aids in the development of biofilms [59, 60]. Additionally, they mediate adherence and internalisation into epithelial cells via β1 intregins [57], can bind to collagen type 1 [61] and interact with other oral microorganisms: *Candida albicans* [62]; *Porphyromonas gingivalis* [63]; and *Actinomyces naeslundii* [60]. Given their critical role in induction of platelet aggregation it is tempting to speculate that *S. gordonii* strains lacking antigen I/II proteins may have reduced virulence in IE due to failure to propagate platelet activation. However, this remains to be confirmed in animal models of IE.

The cariogenic and IE causing bacterium *S. mutans* also produces an antigen I/II adhesin called PAc, P1 or SpaA that has been shown to be involved in platelet aggregation [64]. PAc is a LPXTG cell wall associated protein with significant sequence identity to *S. gordonii* SspA [65]. PAc, like SspA and SspB, has roles in adherence to the salivary pellicle, biofilm formation [66], collagen dependent invasion of dentinal tubules binding [67]. Clinical strains lacking expression of PAc failed to induce aggregation in PRP [64]. Additionally, increasing amounts of anti-PAc serum dose dependently decreased the rate of platelet aggregation but did not abolish it [66]. A recent crystallography study examined the detailed structure of the C-terminal in the context of adherence to the salivary pellicle, specifically the binding of carbohydrate moieties [68], however, little is known about the putative platelet interactive domain of PAc. Notably, while antibody titres against PAc are increased in patients with *S. mutans* IE, PAc did not play a role in IE in a rat model of infection [69]. In contrast, a study examining the role of *S. mutans* exopolysaccharides revealed a substantial decrease in the incidence of IE in rats infected with wildtype *S. mutans* and a mutant lacking production of glucan and fructan polysaccharides [70]. Chia et al. later identified a direct interaction of *S. mutans* Xc rhamnose-glucose polymers (RGPs) with both human and rabbit platelets and showed the resulting platelet aggregation response to be mediated in part by anti-RGP IgGs [71]. Such rhamnose rich polymers are common amongst streptococcci and may represent a conserved mechanism of platelet activation by the *Streptococcus* genus [71].

8. High molecular weight repeat protein

Previous studies revealed that *S. gordonii* DL1 could bind to not only to platelet GPIbα but also GPIIb, the α chain of the fibrinogen binding integrin αIIbβ3 [72]. Further studies identified a large 397 kDa cell wall associated protein designated platelet adherence protein A (PadA) on the surface of *S. gordonii* which interacts with GPIIb [73]. The N-terminal fragment of PadA contains a domain with homology to the A1 domain, the platelet interactive domain, of vWF. This, however, showed no particular affinity for the vWF receptor, GPIbα. An isogenic PadA mutant displayed the same affinity for glycocalicin as wildtype DL1 while binding was significantly reduced in a Hsa mutant [73]. In contrast, platelets adhered to immobilised fragments of the N-terminal region (amino acids 34-690) but not to a smaller fragment (amino acids 34-359) also containing the vWF domain suggesting other sites within the protein contribute to platelet adhesion to PadA [73]. Mutants lacking Hsa bound at wildtype levels to Chinese Hamster Ovary (CHO) cells expressing αIIbβ3 while a PadA mutant displayed significantly reduced adhesion. Additionally, CHO cell adhesion to wildtype bacteria was inhibited by a monoclonal antibody to αIIbβ3 (abciximab) and a fibrinopeptide mimetic, RGDS [73]. Interestingly, platelets adhering to immobilised *S. gordonii* DL1 or specific fragments of PadA underwent dramatic changes in morphology as observed by fluorescent confocal microscopy [74]. Rearrangement of the platelet actin cytoskeleton led filopodia and llamelipodia formation, known as platelet spreading [74]. Platelet spreading is critical for the platelet to withstand shear forces experienced in the vasculature. Similar observations were made for platelet adhesion to fibrinogen, suggesting that PadA mimics the prothrombotic surface of immobilised extracellular matrix proteins. Indeed, protein analysis revealed PadA contains RGD-like regions (RGG, RGT and AGD) that may act as binding sites for αIIbβ3 [74]. These observations have led to the model of *S. gordonii* platelet interactions: Hsa and GspB mediate initial attachment of *S. gordonii* to platelets via GPIbα; PadA provides stabilising interactions via αIIbβ3, causing platelet spreading, so that the growing septic thrombus can resist the turbulent forces within the bloodstream; and SspA and SspB are needed to produce the final aggregation phase that propagates vegetation growth [59].

9. Phage encoded proteins

Human and bacterial evolution is peppered with incidences of viral integration or endogenisation into host genomes. Indeed, when the human genome was sequenced it was found that only 1.5% was composed of defined genes [75, 76]. The remainder, formally referred to as "junk DNA", is now known to contain critical regulatory sequences. Many of these regulatory sequences and indeed genes have been linked to viral origins [77-79]. Bacterial history is also littered with incidences of viral DNA integration. Bacterial viruses are called bacteriophages and in the cases below they confer an advantage to *S. mitis* in the pathogenesis of IE.

Using a transposon generated mutant library of *S. mitis* SF100, two genetic loci were identified as having a role in *S. mitis*-platelet interactions [80]. The first, PblT, is predicted to encode a transmembrane transporter with 12 membrane spanning segments [80]. Its role in *S. mitis*-platelet interactions remains to be to be confirmed. Interestingly, the second locus was demonstrated to be a bacteriophage, SM1, of the *Siphoviridae* family of bacteriophages [81] and is widespread in the microbial population of the oropharynx and saliva as shown in a recent metagenomic study of oral viral communities [82]. Two proteins, PblA and PblB, encoded in the polycistronic operon of this phage were shown to mediate *S. mitis* binding to platelets [80,

83]. PblA and PblB are expressed on the bacterial surface through a novel mechanism whereby the proteins are exported and become associated with bacterial cells via choline residues in their cell wall [84]. While the ability to bind choline residues is found in other streptococcal expressed proteins (*S. pneumoniae* LytA), PblA and PblB bear little homology to previously identified bacterial adhesins [80]. Instead, they are similar to the tail fibre proteins of phage particles [80]. Recently a comprehensive study by Mitchell et al., utilizing linkage specific sialidases, concluded that PblA and PblB bind sialic acid residues on α2-8 linked gangliosides [85]. Consistent with this, platelets express only one such ganglioside, GD3, and specific antibodies to this receptor significantly reduced binding of wild type *S. mitis* SF100 to platelets while a mutant, with already significantly reduced in binding to platelets, remained unaffected [85]. The precise role of this receptor in conventional platelet activation remains to be determined but it has been shown to be upregulated on activated platelets, later becoming internalised and associating with the Src tyrosine kinase, Lyn, and then with FcRγ and leading to increased FcγRIIA expression [86]. How *S. mitis* would propagate platelet activation through this receptor remains to be elucidated.

Interestingly, during the investigation of PblA and PblB, a study revealed that mutation of the bacteriophage lysin gene, *lys*, needed to permeablise cells and release lytic phage particles, caused a reduction in platelet binding greater than that of the $PblA^-/PblB^-$ mutant [84]. When investigated further, the phage lysin was found to bind fibrinogen via the D fragment of the Aα and Bβ chains, and in doing so can mediate an indirect interaction with human platelets through αIIbβ3 [87]. Like PblA and PblB, it is also a choline binding protein but with homology to the choline binding domain of pneumococcal LytA [87]. The fibrinogen interactive domain was localized to amino acids 102-198 [88] and when this polypeptide was preincubated with platelets and *S. mitis* SF100, it significantly extended the lag time to aggregation. Furthermore, in a rat model of endocarditis, co-infection with $PblA^-/PblB^-$ and lys^- mutants led to substantially less inclusion of lys^- *S. mitis* in the vegetations as compared to the tail protein mutant, $PblA^-/PblB^-$. $Lysin_{SM1}$ is considered a multifunctional phage protein, mediating lysis of *S. mitis* in the bacteriophage lytic life cycle, binding to choline residues in the cell wall and binding to fibrinogen, bridging an interaction with human platelets via αIIbβ3 [87], an interaction that is repeated in multiple streptococcal species and considered an important interaction in the pathogenesis of IE (see figure).

10. Secreted products

Bacteria can secrete bioactive molecules that participate in platelet interactions *in trans*, independently of bacterial cell binding. Early studies examining the role of aetiological agents in Kawasaki disease (an inflammatory disease characterised by systemic vasculitis) isolated a strain of *S mitis* (Nm65) whose culture supernatant appeared to induce platelet aggregation in platelet rich plasma [89]. This activity was isolated to a heat labile, 66kDa protein antigen called sm-hPAF (*S. mitis* derived human platelet aggregation factor) [90]. Notably, 'aggregation' was not inhibited by treatment of platelets with prostaglandin E_1 (PGE_1), which increases intracellular cyclic-AMP preventing platelet signalling, or the αIIbβ3 inhibitory peptide (RGDS) and

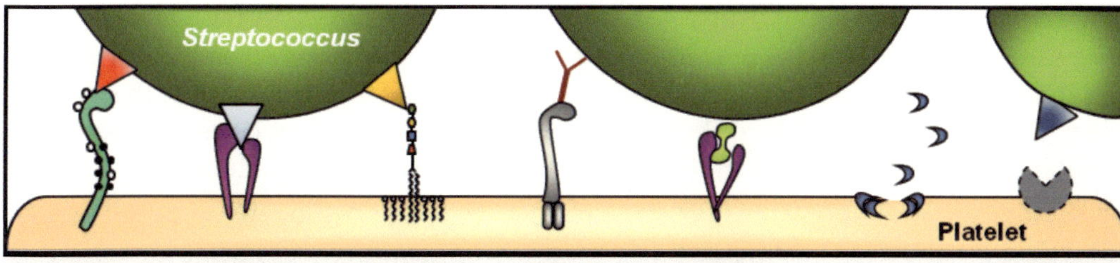

GPIbα	αIIbβ3 (direct)	Ganglioside GD3	IgG - FcγRIIA	Fibrinogen - αIIbβ3 (indirect)	?	Unknown receptors
S. gordonii (Hsa/GspB) *S. sanguinis* (SrpA)	*S. gordonii* (PadA)	*S. mitis* (PblA, PblB)	*S. sanguinis* *S. mitis* *S. mutans* *S. pyogenes* *S. agalactiae* *S. oralis*	*S. agalactiae* (FbsA) *S. mitis* (Lysin$_{SM1}$) *S. pyogenes* (M protein)	*S. mitis* (sm-hPAF/ lectinolysin)	*S. sanguinis* (PAAP) *S. gordonii* (SspA/SspB) *S. mutans* (PAc,RGPs)

Figure 1. Schematic of streptococcal platelet interactions in infective endocarditis.

was considered to induce platelet aggregation via novel mechanism [90]. With developments in our understanding of platelet aggregation, inhibition of platelet signalling and activation by PGE_1 and αIIbβ3 dependency are hallmarks of true platelet aggregation. Sm-hPAF (Nm-65 derived) and lectinolysin (SK597derived) were later purified independently and identified as members of the cholesterol dependent cytolysin (CDC) family of bacterial toxins which form oligomeric lytic pores in erythrocyte membranes [90, 91]. Both lectinolysin and Sm-hPAF possess an additional N-terminal fucose binding domain homologous to an agglutinin from the eel species *Anguilla Anguilla*. Interstingly, lectinolysin was demonstrated to induce pore formation via a mechanism modulated by fucosylated glycan binding to the N-terminal domain [91]. However, this domain did not participate in initial receptor recognition as lysis was detected in the absence of a functional glycan binding domain [91] and additional members of the CDC family lacking this domain, suislysin and pneumolysin, also induced platelet lysis [92]. The role of platelet lysis in IE remains to be established.

11. Streptococcal-platelet interactions — Signalling response

Following platelet activation platelets secrete signalling molecules and platelet agonists from their cytoplasmic granules to recruit and activate nearby platelets. *S. sanguinis* can modulate the platelet response through an unusual interaction whereby a surface associated enzyme can modify secreted platelet agonists. Early studies by Herzberg et al. demonstrated that *S. sanguinis* could hydrolyse exogenous ATP to ADP and this was postulated as a mechanism causing platelet aggregation as a cell free supernatant of *S. sanguinis* preincubated with ATP could induce platelet aggregation almost immediately [93]. Later MacFarlane et al. demonstrated that this ecto-ATPase activity localized to a cell wall fraction of *S. sanguinis* [94]. Fan et al. have recently identified a cell wall anchored ecto-5′ nucleotidase (Nt5e) from *S. sanguinis* which can hydrolyse ATP, ADP and AMP producing adenosine [95]. A mutant lacking Nt5e expression had a shortened lag time to platelet aggregation with no effect on platelet adhesion but, interestingly, had decreased virulence in a rabbit model of IE as compared to the wildtype. This was suggested to be due to the inhibition of professional phagocytes, monocytes and macrophages by adenosine, an anti-inflammatory molecule [95]. In addition, the delay in platelet aggregation may delay the release of platelet microbicidal proteins from their granules thus inhibiting the platelet immune response [95].

As mentioned, platelets spread on *S. gordonii* DL1. While platelet spreading is critical for thrombus stability, dense granule secretion is important for amplification of the platelet response, facilitating activation of nearby platelets, recruiting them to the growing thrombus. Both result from initiation of an intracellular signalling cascade caused by PadA engagement of αIIbβ3 [74]. Interestingly, inhibition of platelet FcγRIIA by a monoclonal antibody (Clone IV.3) prevented both platelet spreading and dense granule secretion [74]. FcγRIIA is an ITAM containing receptor [96]. It has an extracellular domain that interacts with immune complexes and an intracellular domain which is proposed to act as a signalling scaffold allowing recruitment protein kinases and phosphatases. Following platelet adhesion and spreading on *S. gordonii* DL1, immunopercipitation of FcγRIIA and its downstream effectors revealed tyrosine phosphorylation of FcγRIIA, Syk and phospholipase Cγ (PLCγ – an effector of dense granule secretion) [74]. Blockade of FcγRIIA by the antibody IV.3 prevented phosphorylation of FcγRIIA and its downstream effectors while it had no effect on platelet adhesion to *S. gordonii* DL1 demonstrating an essential role in platelet activation and signalling but not in initial attachment to the bacterium.

Similarly, Pampolina et al. examined the phosphorylation state of the FcγRIIA and its downstream effectors during the platelet aggregation response to *S. sanguinis* 2017-78. *S. sanguinis* 2017-78 induced phosphorylation of FcγRIIA, Syk, Linker for activation of T-cells (LAT) and PLCγ 30 seconds after the addition of bacteria to the platelet suspension [97]. This was followed by dephosphorylation during the lag phase and αIIbβ3 and thromboxane dependent rephosphorylation as aggregation proceeded [97]. The MAP kinase Erk was observed to follow the same triphasic phosphorylation profile in response to *S. sanguinis* 2017-78 [98]. The dephosphorylation phase is proposed to be due to the activity of platelet endothelial cell adhesion molecule-1 (PECAM-1), an ITIM containing receptor which recruits the tyrosine phosphatase SHP-1 during the lag phase [97]. Further studies by McNicol et al. highlighted a role for PI3 kinase mediated phosphorylation of Erk in response to *S. sanguinis* 2017-78 [99]. PI3 kinase is found downstream of FcγRIIA and GPIb and upstream of the GTPase Rap1b, critical for αIIbβ3 activation [100, 101].

12. Streptococcal-platelet interactions — Immunological response

When bacteria enter the bloodstream they are recognised by soluble elements of the immune system. These soluble elements, specifically immunoglobulins and complement proteins can bind to their respective receptors on professional immune cells and platelets forming indirect bridging interactions. As most bacteria causing infective endocarditis are in fact lifelong or transient residents of the host, most of the population inherently produce a humoral immune response to these bacteria.

The role of IgG in platelet bacterial interactions has been extensively studied and reaffirmed repeatedly in the literature [28, 102-105]. Its role was first confirmed by Sullam et al. who demonstrated that plasma components other than fibrinogen (a cofactor for ADP induced activation) was required for *S. sanguinis* M99 and *S. salivarius* D1 induced platelet aggregation [104]. Additionally, blockade of the platelet low affinity IgG receptor, FcγRIIA, with a monoclonal antibody IV.3 completely inhibited platelet aggregation in response to these bacteria [104]. In fact, inhibition of FcγRIIA has inhibited all bacterial induced aggregation when examined, even in the absence of IgG interactions consolidating its role in platelet activation by bacteria [30, 74, 84, 97, 102, 106-108]. The nature of these antibodies, however, remains more complex as some bacteria require strain specific [107], species specific or, minimally, group specific antibodies [105]. Many conserved structural entities of bacteria elicit antibody responses e.g., peptidoglycan and lipoteichoic acids. Therefore, it is plausible that specific subclasses of antibody cross react between streptococcal species while others recognise species and strain specific antigens. Indeed, while IgG1 and IgG3 largely bind protein antigens, IgG2 binds to carbohydrate antigens [109]. Antibody levels in the host were first thought to determine the variable lag times observed between donors however this could not be established and led to investigations of other plasma proteins mediating platelet-bacterial interactions. Additionally, in a study of aggregating and non aggregating strains of *S. sanguinis* and *S. gordonii*, significant correlation between the levels of specific antibody and the propensity to induce aggregation was observed, but this was not true for all donors [105]. Notably, non aggregating strains and their non aggregating donor pairs were shown to have similar levels of strain specific antibody to donors who did support platelet aggregation [105]. This was not explained by polymorphisms in FcγRIIA and thus is most likely a result of secondary interactions with other receptors, differences in receptor number or polymorphisms therein but this remains to be investigated.

The complement system is a series of proteins that bind to bacteria in a step wise fashion and culminate in the formation of an oligomeric pore, the membrane attack complex, which lyses the targeted bacterium. Roles for complement in bacterial-platelet interactions have been demonstrated in *Staphylococcal aureus* and *S. sanguinis* [102, 107, 110]. The lag time to aggregation in platelet rich plasma (PRP) in response to *S. sanguinis* 7863 is 7-19 minutes [111] and this variation was correlated to the rate of assembly of the C5b-9 complex on the surface of the bacteria as detected by flow cytometry [110]. Accordingly, the lag time to aggregation using bacterial cells preincubated with plasma before addition to PRP could be progressively shortened with extension of the incubation time [110]. Complement activation can be triggered by antigen-antibody complexes (classical pathway) or by binding of specific complement proteins (alternative pathway) or mannose binding protein (lectin pathway) to the microbial surface. *S. sanguinis* 7863 induced the alternative pathway, as shown by direct and Mg2+ dependent binding of complement protein C3 to the surface of the bacterium [110]. Inactivation of complement by cobra venom or heat treatment abolished aggregation [110] suggesting that other interactions, namely IgG with FcγRIIA, were not sufficient to produce aggregation alone. It is not known precisely how complement activation triggers platelet activation but it is possible that there is a threshold of bacterial-platelet interactions (capable of inducing strong or weak signals) which much be surpassed before triggering platelet aggregation however this remains to be investigated.

While previous reports examined platelet secretion in terms of end stage platelet activation, namely aggregation and spreading, a number of studies exist investigating the role of platelet secretion in the context of platelet immunology. In addition to platelet agonists, platelet granules contain bacteriocidal proteins and cytokines. A recent study by McNicol et al. demonstrated platelet activity in the form of signalling and secretion in the absence of platelet aggregation. They examined platelet secretion of soluble inflammatory mediators (Platelet factor 4, RANTES, sCD40L, platelet derived growth factor) in response to a number of *S. sanguinis* and *S. gordonii* strains and paired these with their platelet aggregation responses. All strains triggered secretion of cytokines irrespective of the platelet aggregation response but only 1 strain (*S. sanguinis* 2017-78) triggered release of sCD62p [99]. For *S. sanguinis* 2017-78 cytokine secretion was independent of thromboxane production and aggregation. Interestingly this secretion response was inhibited by low doses of epinephrine while aggregation and protein phosphorylation cascades mentioned previously were enhanced [99]. The inhibition of platelet activation by epinephrine has not been noted in response to any other platelet agonists and adds another layer of complexity to bacterial induced platelet activation. It will be interesting to examine the contribution of individual platelet-bacterial interactions this novel platelet activation in the future.

13. Conclusion

The overall role of platelet activation in response to circulating bacteria and IE is controversial but recent studies have linked platelet activation to the ability of bacteria to resist antibiotics [112]. This is consistent with the concept that, in activating platelets, bacteria prevent infiltration by antibiotics (or recognition by the immune system). It is likely that the initial adhesion events occur independently of platelet activation and thus make suitable targets in the prevention of IE. In contrast, as the ability to induce platelet aggregation (activation) *in vitro* contributes to the virulence and persistence of the organism in infective endocarditis animal models [87, 95], the pathways of platelet aggregation are targets of future IE therapies. Consistent with this, a recent study has examined the effect of antiplatelet drug Reopro (abciximab) in the treatment of sepsis in mice [113] and the use of cyclooxygenase inhibitors, e.g. aspirin and inbuprofen continue to be investigated [114-117]. Critically, future therapies must balance immune function and haemostatic function of platelets making thorough understanding of platelet-bacterial interactions and bacterial induced platelet activation essential for future drug development.

Author details

Dorothea Tilley and Steven W. Kerrigan

School of Pharmacy & Molecular and Cellular Therapeutics, Royal College of Surgeons in Ireland, Dublin, Ireland

References

[1] Ruggeri, Z.M., *Platelet adhesion under flow.* Microcirculation, 2009. 16(1): p. 58-83.

[2] Durack, D.T. and P.B. Beeson, *Experimental bacterial endocarditis. I. Colonization of a sterile vegetation.* Br J Exp Pathol, 1972. 53(1): p. 44-9.

[3] Yvorchuk, K.J. and K.L. Chan, *Application of transthoracic and transesophageal echocardiography in the diagnosis and management of infective endocarditis.* J Am Soc Echocardiogr, 1994. 7(3 Pt 1): p. 294-308.

[4] Wilson, W., et al., *Prevention of infective endocarditis: guidelines from the American Heart Association: a guideline from the American Heart Association Rheumatic Fever, Endocarditis, and Kawasaki Disease Committee, Council on Cardiovascular Disease in the Young, and the Council on Clinical Cardiology, Council on Cardiovascular Surgery and Anesthesia, and the Quality of Care and Outcomes Research Interdisciplinary Working Group.* Circulation, 2007. 116(15): p. 1736-54.

[5] Durack, D.T. and P.B. Beeson, *Experimental bacterial endocarditis. II. Survival of a bacteria in endocardial vegetations.* Br J Exp Pathol, 1972. 53(1): p. 50-3.

[6] Schierholz, J.M., J. Beuth, and G. Pulverer, *"Difficult to treat infections" pharmacokinetic and pharmacodynamic factors--a review.* Acta Microbiol Immunol Hung, 2000. 47(1): p. 1-8.

[7] Fowler, V.G., Jr., et al., *Staphylococcus aureus endocarditis: a consequence of medical progress.* JAMA, 2005. 293(24): p. 3012-21.

[8] Tleyjeh, I.M., et al., *Temporal trends in infective endocarditis: a population-based study in Olmsted County, Minnesota.* JAMA, 2005. 293(24): p. 3022-8.

[9] Douglas, C.W., et al., *Identity of viridans streptococci isolated from cases of infective endocarditis.* J Med Microbiol, 1993. 39(3): p. 179-82.

[10] Andrews, R.K., et al., *Glycoprotein Ib-IX-V.* Int J Biochem Cell Biol, 2003. 35(8): p. 1170-4.

[11] Canobbio, I., C. Balduini, and M. Torti, *Signalling through the platelet glycoprotein Ib-V-IX complex.* Cell Signal, 2004. 16(12): p. 1329-44.

[12] Savage, B., E. Saldivar, and Z.M. Ruggeri, *Initiation of platelet adhesion by arrest onto fibrinogen or translocation on von Willebrand factor.* Cell, 1996. 84(2): p. 289-97.

[13] Santoro, S.A., *Identification of a 160,000 dalton platelet membrane protein that mediates the initial divalent cation-dependent adhesion of platelets to collagen.* Cell, 1986. 46(6): p. 913-20.

[14] Kunicki, T.J., et al., *The human fibroblast class II extracellular matrix receptor mediates platelet adhesion to collagen and is identical to the platelet glycoprotein Ia-IIa complex.* J Biol Chem, 1988. 263(10): p. 4516-9.

[15] Nieuwenhuis, H.K., et al., *Human blood platelets showing no response to collagen fail to express surface glycoprotein Ia.* Nature, 1985. 318(6045): p. 470-2.

[16] Varga-Szabo, D., I. Pleines, and B. Nieswandt, *Cell adhesion mechanisms in platelets.* Arterioscler Thromb Vasc Biol, 2008. 28(3): p. 403-12.

[17] Savage, B., F. Almus-Jacobs, and Z.M. Ruggeri, *Specific synergy of multiple substrate-receptor interactions in platelet thrombus formation under flow.* Cell, 1998. 94(5): p. 657-66.

[18] Plow, E.F., S.E. D'Souza, and M.H. Ginsberg, *Ligand binding to GPIIb-IIIa: a status report.* Semin Thromb Hemost, 1992. 18(3): p. 324-32.

[19] Hartwig, J.H., *Platelet Structure,* A.D. Michelson, Editor 2002, Academic Press: London. p. 37-52.

[20] Semple, J.W., J.E. Italiano, Jr., and J. Freedman, *Platelets and the immune continuum.* Nat Rev Immunol, 2011. 11(4): p. 264-74.

[21] Krijgsveld, J., et al., *Thrombocidins, microbicidal proteins from human blood platelets, are C-terminal deletion products of CXC chemokines.* J Biol Chem, 2000. 275(27): p. 20374-81.

[22] Cognasse, F., et al., *Evidence of Toll-like receptor molecules on human platelets.* Immunol Cell Biol, 2005. 83(2): p. 196-8.

[23] Shiraki, R., et al., *Expression of Toll-like receptors on human platelets.* Thromb Res, 2004. 113(6): p. 379-85.

[24] McNicol, A. and S.J. Israels, *Beyond hemostasis: the role of platelets in inflammation, malignancy and infection.* Cardiovasc Hematol Disord Drug Targets, 2008. 8(2): p. 99-117.

[25] Clemetson, K.J., et al., *Functional expression of CCR1, CCR3, CCR4, and CXCR4 chemokine receptors on human platelets.* Blood, 2000. 96(13): p. 4046-54.

[26] Clemetson, K.J. and J.M. Clemetson, *Platelet Receptors,* in *Platelets,* A.D. Michelson, Editor 2007, Academic Press: London. p. 126-143.

[27] Cosgrove, L.J., et al., *CR3 receptor on platelets and its role in the prostaglandin metabolic pathway.* Immunol Cell Biol, 1987. 65 (Pt 6): p. 453-60.

[28] Ford, I. and C.W. Douglas, *The role of platelets in infective endocarditis.* Platelets, 1997. 8(5): p. 285-94.

[29] Fitzgerald, J.R., T.J. Foster, and D. Cox, *The interaction of bacterial pathogens with platelets.* Nat Rev Microbiol, 2006. 4(6): p. 445-57.

[30] Kerrigan, S.W., et al., *A role for glycoprotein Ib in Streptococcus sanguis-induced platelet aggregation.* Blood, 2002. 100(2): p. 509-16.

[31] O'Brien, L., et al., *Multiple mechanisms for the activation of human platelet aggregation by Staphylococcus aureus: roles for the clumping factors ClfA and ClfB, the serine-aspartate repeat protein SdrE and protein A.* Mol Microbiol, 2002. 44(4): p. 1033-44.

[32] Herzberg, M.C., et al., *Platelet-interactive products of Streptococcus sanguis protoplasts.* Infect Immun, 1990. 58(12): p. 4117-25.

[33] Erickson, P.R. and M.C. Herzberg, *Evidence for the covalent linkage of carbohydrate polymers to a glycoprotein from Streptococcus sanguis.* J Biol Chem, 1993. 268(32): p. 23780-3.

[34] Upreti, R.K., M. Kumar, and V. Shankar, *Bacterial glycoproteins: functions, biosynthesis and applications.* Proteomics, 2003. 3(4): p. 363-79.

[35] Soberay, A.H., et al., *Responses of platelets to strains of streptococcus sanguis: findings in healthy subjects, Bernard-Soulier, Glanzmann's, and collagen-unresponsive patients.* Thromb Haemost, 1987. 57(2): p. 222-5.

[36] Gong, K., et al., *Platelet receptors for the Streptococcus sanguis adhesin and aggregation-associated antigens are distinguished by anti-idiotypical monoclonal antibodies.* Infect Immun, 1995. 63(9): p. 3628-33.

[37] Erickson, P.R. and M.C. Herzberg, *Purification and partial characterization of a 65-kDa platelet aggregation-associated protein antigen from the surface of Streptococcus sanguis.* J Biol Chem, 1990. 265(24): p. 14080-7.

[38] Erickson, P.R., M.C. Herzberg, and G. Tierney, *Cross-reactive immunodeterminants on Streptococcus sanguis and collagen. Predicting a structural motif of platelet-interactive domains.* J Biol Chem, 1992. 267(14): p. 10018-23.

[39] Erickson, P.R. and M.C. Herzberg, *The Streptococcus sanguis platelet aggregation-associated protein. Identification and characterization of the minimal platelet-interactive domain.* J Biol Chem, 1993. 268(3): p. 1646-9.

[40] Herzberg, M.C., et al., *Oral streptococci and cardiovascular disease: searching for the platelet aggregation-associated protein gene and mechanisms of Streptococcus sanguis-induced thrombosis.* J Periodontol, 2005. 76(11 Suppl): p. 2101-5.

[41] Plummer, C., et al., *A serine-rich glycoprotein of Streptococcus sanguis mediates adhesion to platelets via GPIb.* Br J Haematol, 2005. 129(1): p. 101-9.

[42] Bensing, B.A., J.A. Lopez, and P.M. Sullam, *The Streptococcus gordonii surface proteins GspB and Hsa mediate binding to sialylated carbohydrate epitopes on the platelet membrane glycoprotein Ibalpha.* Infect Immun, 2004. 72(11): p. 6528-37.

[43] Takamatsu, D., et al., *Binding of the Streptococcus gordonii surface glycoproteins GspB and Hsa to specific carbohydrate structures on platelet membrane glycoprotein Ibalpha.* Mol Microbiol, 2005. 58(2): p. 380-92.

[44] Bensing, B.A. and P.M. Sullam, *An accessory sec locus of Streptococcus gordonii is required for export of the surface protein GspB and for normal levels of binding to human platelets.* Mol Microbiol, 2002. 44(4): p. 1081-94.

[45] Wu, H. and P.M. Fives-Taylor, *Identification of dipeptide repeats and a cell wall sorting signal in the fimbriae-associated adhesin, Fap1, of Streptococcus parasanguis.* Mol Microbiol, 1999. 34(5): p. 1070-81.

[46] Takahashi, Y., et al., *Functional analysis of the Streptococcus gordonii DL1 sialic acid-binding adhesin and its essential role in bacterial binding to platelets.* Infect Immun, 2004. 72(7): p. 3876-82.

[47] Takahashi, Y., et al., *Identification and characterization of hsa, the gene encoding the sialic acid-binding adhesin of Streptococcus gordonii DL1.* Infect Immun, 2002. 70(3): p. 1209-18.

[48] Stephenson, A.E., et al., *The Fap1 fimbrial adhesin is a glycoprotein: antibodies specific for the glycan moiety block the adhesion of Streptococcus parasanguis in an in vitro tooth model.* Mol Microbiol, 2002. 43(1): p. 147-57.

[49] Wu, H., et al., *Isolation and characterization of Fap1, a fimbriae-associated adhesin of Streptococcus parasanguis FW213.* Mol Microbiol, 1998. 28(3): p. 487-500.

[50] Froeliger, E.H. and P. Fives-Taylor, *Streptococcus parasanguis fimbria-associated adhesin fap1 is required for biofilm formation.* Infect Immun, 2001. 69(4): p. 2512-9.

[51] Wu, H., M. Zeng, and P. Fives-Taylor, *The glycan moieties and the N-terminal polypeptide backbone of a fimbria-associated adhesin, Fap1, play distinct roles in the biofilm development of Streptococcus parasanguinis.* Infect Immun, 2007. 75(5): p. 2181-8.

[52] van Sorge, N.M., et al., *The group B streptococcal serine-rich repeat 1 glycoprotein mediates penetration of the blood-brain barrier.* J Infect Dis, 2009. 199(10): p. 1479-87.

[53] Shivshankar, P., et al., *The Streptococcus pneumoniae adhesin PsrP binds to Keratin 10 on lung cells.* Mol Microbiol, 2009. 73(4): p. 663-79.

[54] Pyburn, T.M., et al., *A structural model for binding of the serine-rich repeat adhesin GspB to host carbohydrate receptors.* PLoS Pathog, 2011. 7(7): p. e1002112.

[55] Andrews, R.K., M.C. Berndt, and J. Lopez Gorge, *The Glycoprotein Ib-IX-V Complex*, in *Platelets*, A.D. Michelson, Editor 2002, Academic Press: London. p. 145-163.

[56] Kerrigan, S.W., et al., *Role of Streptococcus gordonii surface proteins SspA/SspB and Hsa in platelet function.* Infect Immun, 2007. 75(12): p. 5740-7.

[57] Nobbs, A.H., et al., *Adherence and internalization of Streptococcus gordonii by epithelial cells involves beta1 integrin recognition by SspA and SspB (antigen I/II family) polypeptides.* Cell Microbiol, 2007. 9(1): p. 65-83.

[58] Jenkinson, H.F. and D.R. Demuth, *Structure, function and immunogenicity of streptococcal antigen I/II polypeptides.* Mol Microbiol, 1997. 23(2): p. 183-90.

[59] Jakubovics, N.S., et al., *Functions of cell surface-anchored antigen I/II family and Hsa polypeptides in interactions of Streptococcus gordonii with host receptors.* Infect Immun, 2005. 73(10): p. 6629-38.

[60] Jakubovics, N.S., et al., *Differential binding specificities of oral streptococcal antigen I/II family adhesins for human or bacterial ligands.* Mol Microbiol, 2005. 55(5): p. 1591-605.

[61] Heddle, C., et al., *Host collagen signal induces antigen I/II adhesin and invasin gene expression in oral Streptococcus gordonii.* Mol Microbiol, 2003. 50(2): p. 597-607.

[62] Egland, P.G., L.D. Du, and P.E. Kolenbrander, *Identification of independent Streptococcus gordonii SspA and SspB functions in coaggregation with Actinomyces naeslundii.* Infect Immun, 2001. 69(12): p. 7512-6.

[63] Demuth, D.R., et al., *Discrete protein determinant directs the species-specific adherence of Porphyromonas gingivalis to oral streptococci.* Infect Immun, 2001. 69(9): p. 5736-41.

[64] Matsumoto-Nakano, M., et al., *Contribution of cell surface protein antigen c of Streptococcus mutans to platelet aggregation.* Oral Microbiol Immunol, 2009. 24(5): p. 427-30.

[65] Demuth, D.R., et al., *Tandem genes encode cell-surface polypeptides SspA and SspB which mediate adhesion of the oral bacterium Streptococcus gordonii to human and bacterial receptors.* Mol Microbiol, 1996. 20(2): p. 403-13.

[66] Pecharki, D., et al., *Involvement of antigen I/II surface proteins in Streptococcus mutans and Streptococcus intermedius biofilm formation.* Oral Microbiol Immunol, 2005. 20(6): p. 366-71.

[67] Love, R.M., M.D. McMillan, and H.F. Jenkinson, *Invasion of dentinal tubules by oral streptococci is associated with collagen recognition mediated by the antigen I/II family of polypeptides.* Infect Immun, 1997. 65(12): p. 5157-64.

[68] Larson, M.R., et al., *Crystal structure of the C-terminal region of Streptococcus mutans antigen I/II and characterization of salivary agglutinin adherence domains.* J Biol Chem, 2011. 286(24): p. 21657-66.

[69] Ryd, M., et al., *Streptococcus mutans major adhesion surface protein, P1 (I/II), does not contribute to attachment to valvular vegetations or to the development of endocarditis in a rat model.* Arch Oral Biol, 1996. 41(10): p. 999-1002.

[70] Munro, C.L. and F.L. Macrina, *Sucrose-derived exopolysaccharides of Streptococcus mutans V403 contribute to infectivity in endocarditis.* Mol Microbiol, 1993. 8(1): p. 133-42.

[71] Chia, J.S., et al., *Platelet aggregation induced by serotype polysaccharides from Streptococcus mutans.* Infect Immun, 2004. 72(5): p. 2605-17.

[72] Yajima, A., Y. Takahashi, and K. Konishi, *Identification of platelet receptors for the Streptococcus gordonii DL1 sialic acid-binding adhesin.* Microbiol Immunol, 2005. 49(8): p. 795-800.

[73] Petersen, H.J., et al., *Human platelets recognize a novel surface protein, PadA, on Streptococcus gordonii through a unique interaction involving fibrinogen receptor GPIIbIIIa.* Infect Immun, 2010. 78(1): p. 413-22.

[74] Keane, C., et al., *Mechanism of outside-in {alpha}IIb{beta}3-mediated activation of human platelets by the colonizing Bacterium, Streptococcus gordonii.* Arterioscler Thromb Vasc Biol, 2010. 30(12): p. 2408-15.

[75] Human Genome Sequencing, C., *Finishing the euchromatic sequence of the human genome.* Nature, 2004. 431(7011): p. 931-945.

[76] Lander, E.S., et al., *Initial sequencing and analysis of the human genome.* Nature, 2001. 409(6822): p. 860-921.

[77] Blaise, S., et al., *Genomewide screening for fusogenic human endogenous retrovirus envelopes identifies syncytin 2, a gene conserved on primate evolution.* Proc Natl Acad Sci U S A, 2003. 100(22): p. 13013-8.

[78] Blond, J.L., et al., *An envelope glycoprotein of the human endogenous retrovirus HERV-W is expressed in the human placenta and fuses cells expressing the type D mammalian retrovirus receptor.* J Virol, 2000. 74(7): p. 3321-9.

[79] Mi, S., et al., *Syncytin is a captive retroviral envelope protein involved in human placental morphogenesis.* Nature, 2000. 403(6771): p. 785-9.

[80] Bensing, B.A., C.E. Rubens, and P.M. Sullam, *Genetic loci of Streptococcus mitis that mediate binding to human platelets.* Infect Immun, 2001. 69(3): p. 1373-80.

[81] Siboo, I.R., B.A. Bensing, and P.M. Sullam, *Genomic organization and molecular characterization of SM1, a temperate bacteriophage of Streptococcus mitis.* J Bacteriol, 2003. 185(23): p. 6968-75.

[82] Willner, D., et al., *Metagenomic detection of phage-encoded platelet-binding factors in the human oral cavity.* Proc Natl Acad Sci U S A, 2010. 108 Suppl 1: p. 4547-53.

[83] Bensing, B.A., I.R. Siboo, and P.M. Sullam, *Proteins PblA and PblB of Streptococcus mitis, which promote binding to human platelets, are encoded within a lysogenic bacteriophage.* Infect Immun, 2001. 69(10): p. 6186-92.

[84] Mitchell, J., et al., *Mechanism of cell surface expression of the Streptococcus mitis platelet binding proteins PblA and PblB.* Mol Microbiol, 2007. 64(3): p. 844-57.

[85] Mitchell, J. and P.M. Sullam, *Streptococcus mitis phage-encoded adhesins mediate attachment to {alpha}2-8-linked sialic acid residues on platelet membrane gangliosides.* Infect Immun, 2009. 77(8): p. 3485-90.

[86] Martini, F., et al., *Involvement of GD3 in platelet activation. A novel association with Fcgamma receptor.* Biochim Biophys Acta, 2002. 1583(3): p. 297-304.

[87] Seo, H.S., et al., *Bacteriophage lysin mediates the binding of streptococcus mitis to human platelets through interaction with fibrinogen.* PLoS Pathog, 2010. 6(8): p. e1001047.

[88] Seo, H.S. and P.M. Sullam, *Characterization of the fibrinogen binding domain of bacteriophage lysin from Streptococcus mitis.* Infect Immun, 2011. 79(9): p. 3518-26.

[89] Ohkuni, H., et al., *Biologically active extracellular products of oral viridans streptococci and the aetiology of Kawasaki disease.* J Med Microbiol, 1993. 39(5): p. 352-62.

[90] Ohkuni, H., et al., *Purification and partial characterization of a novel human platelet aggregation factor in the extracellular products of Streptococcus mitis, strain Nm-65.* FEMS Immunol Med Microbiol, 1997. 17(2): p. 121-9.

[91] Farrand, S., et al., *Characterization of a streptococcal cholesterol-dependent cytolysin with a lewis y and b specific lectin domain.* Biochemistry, 2008. 47(27): p. 7097-107.

[92] Ohkuni H, Nagamune H, Ozaki N, Tabata A, Todome Y, Watanabe Y, Takahashi H, Ohkura K, Kourai H, Ohtsuka H, Fischetti VA, Zabriskie JB. Characterization of recombinant Streptococcus mitis-derived human platelet aggregation factor. APMIS 2012 Jan;120(1):56-71

[93] Herzberg, M.C. and K.L. Brintzenhofe, *ADP-like platelet aggregation activity generated by viridans streptococci incubated with exogenous ATP.* Infect Immun, 1983. 40(1): p. 120-5.

[94] MacFarlane, G.D., et al., *Evidence for an ecto-ATPase on the cell wall of Streptococcus sanguis.* Oral Microbiol Immunol, 1994. 9(3): p. 180-5.

[95] Fan, J., et al., *Ecto-5'-nucleotidase: a candidate virulence factor in Streptococcus sanguinis experimental endocarditis.* PLoS One, 2012. 7(6): p. e38059.

[96] Van den Herik-Oudijk, I.E., et al., *Identification of signaling motifs within human Fc gamma RIIa and Fc gamma RIIb isoforms.* Blood, 1995. 85(8): p. 2202-11.

[97] Pampolina, C. and A. McNicol, *Streptococcus sanguis-induced platelet activation involves two waves of tyrosine phosphorylation mediated by FcgammaRIIA and alphaIIbbeta3.* Thromb Haemost, 2005. 93(5): p. 932-9.

[98] Abdulrehman AY, Jackson EC, McNicol A. Platelet activation by Streptococcus sanguinis is accompanied by MAP kinase phosphorylation. Platelets 2013;24(1):6-14

[99] McNicol, A., et al., *Streptococcus sanguinis-induced cytokine release from platelets.* J Thromb Haemost, 2011. 9(10): p. 2038-49.

[100] Lova, P., et al., *A selective role for phosphatidylinositol 3,4,5-trisphosphate in the Gi-dependent activation of platelet Rap1B.* J Biol Chem, 2003. 278(1): p. 131-8.

[101] Munday, A.D., M.C. Berndt, and C.A. Mitchell, *Phosphoinositide 3-kinase forms a complex with platelet membrane glycoprotein Ib-IX-V complex and 14-3-3zeta.* Blood, 2000. 96(2): p. 577-84.

[102] Loughman, A., et al., *Roles for fibrinogen, immunoglobulin and complement in platelet activation promoted by Staphylococcus aureus clumping factor A.* Mol Microbiol, 2005. 57(3): p. 804-18.

[103] Kerrigan, S.W., et al., *Molecular basis for Staphylococcus aureus-mediated platelet aggregate formation under arterial shear in vitro.* Arterioscler Thromb Vasc Biol, 2008. 28(2): p. 335-40.

[104] Sullam, P.M., G.A. Jarvis, and F.H. Valone, *Role of immunoglobulin G in platelet aggregation by viridans group streptococci.* Infect Immun, 1988. 56(11): p. 2907-11.

[105] McNicol, A., et al., *A role for immunoglobulin G in donor-specific Streptococcus sanguis-induced platelet aggregation.* Thromb Haemost, 2006. 95(2): p. 288-93.

[106] Keane, C., et al., *Invasive Streptococcus pneumoniae trigger platelet activation via Toll-like receptor 2.* J Thromb Haemost, 2010. 8(12): p. 2757-65.

[107] Ford, I., et al., *The role of immunoglobulin G and fibrinogen in platelet aggregation by Streptococcus sanguis.* Br J Haematol, 1997. 97(4): p. 737-46.

[108] Byrne, M.F., et al., *Helicobacter pylori binds von Willebrand factor and interacts with GPIb to induce platelet aggregation.* Gastroenterology, 2003. 124(7): p. 1846-54.

[109] Hammarstrom, L. and C.I. Smith, *IgG subclasses in bacterial infections.* Monogr Allergy, 1986. 19: p. 122-33.

[110] Ford, I., et al., *Evidence for the involvement of complement proteins in platelet aggregation by Streptococcus sanguis NCTC 7863.* Br J Haematol, 1996. 94(4): p. 729-39.

[111] Ford, I., et al., *Mechanisms of platelet aggregation by Streptococcus sanguis, a causative organism in infective endocarditis.* Br J Haematol, 1993. 84(1): p. 95-100.

[112] Jung, C.J., et al., *Platelets enhance biofilm formation and resistance of endocarditis-inducing streptococci on the injured heart valve.* J Infect Dis, 2012. 205(7): p. 1066-75.

[113] Sharron, M., et al., *Platelets Induce Apoptosis during Sepsis in a Contact-Dependent Manner That Is Inhibited by GPIIb/IIIa Blockade.* PLoS One, 2012. 7(7): p. e41549.

[114] Kupferwasser, L.I., et al., *Salicylic acid attenuates virulence in endovascular infections by targeting global regulatory pathways in Staphylococcus aureus.* J Clin Invest, 2003. 112(2): p. 222-33.

http://dx.doi.org/10.5772/55912

[115] Sedlacek, M., et al., *Aspirin treatment is associated with a significantly decreased risk of Staphylococcus aureus bacteremia in hemodialysis patients with tunneled catheters.* Am J Kidney Dis, 2007. 49(3): p. 401-8.

[116] Chan, K.-L., et al., *Effect of Long-Term Aspirin Use on Embolic Events in Infective Endocarditis.* Clinical Infectious Diseases, 2008. 46(1): p. 37-41.

[117] Bernard, G.R., et al., *The effects of ibuprofen on the physiology and survival of patients with sepsis. The Ibuprofen in Sepsis Study Group.* N Engl J Med, 1997. 336(13): p. 912-8.

Chapter 3

Platelet Bacterial Interactions in the Pathogenesis of Infective Endocarditis — Part II: The Staphylococcus

Steven W. Kerrigan

Additional information is available at the end of the chapter

http://dx.doi.org/10.5772/55911

1. Introduction

Infective Endocarditis is a microbial infection characterised by the presence of septic vegetations on the surface of the endocardium (Moreillon and Que, 2004). Infection most commonly occurs on the heart valves that has been damaged by congenital defects such as previous disease or trauma (Durack, 1995). As a result these sites have the ability to generate turbulent blood flow which in turn can cause damage to inner most lining of the blood vessels, the endothelium, which causes surface damage leading to exposure of underlying matrix protein (Ruggeri, 2009). Once exposed this highly thrombogenic surface leads to rapid platelet deposition and the formation of a fibrin network. Circulating bacteria from a transient bacteremia in turn binds to this sterile platelet fibrin nidus which allows a secondary accumulation of platelets that encase the bacteria leading to stable thrombus formation (Moreillon and Que, 2004).

Despite improvements in medical and surgical therapy, invasive staphylococcal disease causing infective endocarditis is still associated with a severe prognosis and remains a significant therapeutic challenge. Once a disease primarily affecting younger patients presenting with rheumatic heart disease, modern times see a significant increase in newer 'at risk' categories including patients with long term indwelling central venous catheters, patients undergoing haemodialysis and invasive intravascular procedures such as arthroplasty, immunocompromized patients and intraveneous drug abusers (Thuny et al., 2012). Treatment of infective endocarditis usually requires a multidisciplinary approach involving specialists in infectious disease, cardiologists and cardiac surgeons. Current treatment regimes consist of aggressive prolonged antibiotic therapy, frequently combined with surgery (Prendergast and Tornos, 2010, Wilson et al., 2007). Prolonged antibiotic use is often less than successful as 40% of patients relapse within 2 months of finishing clinically effective therapy.

Furthermore, prolonged exposure to antibiotics leads to a greater risk of adding to the global problem of multiple antibiotic resistant strains of bacteria. Surgery is a costly and risky alternative, however necessary in up to 47% of patients (Castillo et al., 2000, Murdoch et al., 2009). In many cases surgery is not preferable due to risks associated with cardiac failure, further spread of infection leading to persistent sepsis due to surgical removal of an infected thrombus and/or life threatening embolisation (Jault et al., 1997, Heiro et al., 2000, Thuny et al., 2012, Remadi et al., 2007).

2. The Staphylococcus

Staphylococcus aureus is a gram positive pathogen that continues to cause a significant number of community-acquired and nosocomial infections. It is a normal commensal of the human body and usually lives in harmony with its host without causing symptoms. Its primary habitat is the anterior nares in 20% of the population and is transiently associated with the rest (Foster, 2009). The success of *S. aureus* as an opportunistic pathogen is due in part to its expression of a wide array of microbial surface components recognising adhesive matrix molecules (MSCRAMM's) (Patti et al., 1994). Using these MSCRAMM's *S. aureus* uses a multitude of mechanisms to attach either directly or indirectly to host cells including platelets (O'Brien et al., 2002, Kerrigan et al., 2008, Miajlovic et al., 2010, Fitzgerald et al., 2006, Pawar et al., 2004, George et al., 2006). It is for this reason that *S. aureus* is now the most common and most virulent etiologic pathogen in infective endocarditis.

3. Platelets play a critical role in thrombosis and haemostasis

Platelets are small anucleate cell fragments of the larger haematopoietic precursor cell, the megakaryocyte (Thon and Italiano, 2010) and are crucial mediators of haemostasis. Platelets have no control over gene expression as they do not possess a nucleus however they have got limited capabilities in translational protein synthesis (Lindemann et al., 2001b). The primary role of platelets in haemostasis is to police the integrity of the endothelium to prevent blood loss (Nieswandt et al., 2009). Platelets circulate close to the endothelial cell surface at high shear as individual entities that ordinarily do not interact with any other cell types. A transition from this resting state to an activated state can be rapidly initiated if platelets are exposed to an appropriate stimulus. Disruption of the endothelial cell lining due to trauma or injury to the vascular endothelium platelets rapidly accumulate at the site of injury (Gawaz et al., 2005). Recruitment is a highly controlled event that is initiated by the adhesive interaction between the exposed extracellular matrix proteins in damaged endothelium and specific membrane receptors on the platelet (Tabuchi and Kuebler, 2008). Collagen (Santoro and Zutter, 1995), vonWillebrand factor (vWf) (Ruggeri, 1999), fibronectin (Savage et al., 1998, Kasirer-Friede et al., 2007) and thrombospondin (Jurk et al., 2003) constitute the exposed matrix proteins at the site of injury. Athough plasma proteins such as fibrinogen/fibrin and vitronectin are not

http://dx.doi.org/10.5772/55911

synthesized by endothelial cells they can bind to exposed matrix proteins and increase adhesiveness at the damaged site (Ruggeri et al., 2006, Ruggeri and Mendolicchio, 2007).

Platelets express a vast array of membrane receptors that play a critical role in recognition of matrix proteins. The initial interaction of platelets with the injured vessel wall occurs between GPIbα and immobilised vonWillebrand factor (Chesterman and Berndt, 1986). This interaction initiates the tethering of circulating platelets to the vessel wall. Platelets typically 'roll' over the vWf in the direction of flow driven by shear forces experienced by the vasculature (Ruggeri, 2009). A loss of interaction between GPIb and vWf on one side of the platelet leads to the formation of another GPIb-vWf interaction on the other side of the platelet which gives rise to a rolling phenomenon. This rolling mechanism is critical to slowing down the platelet long enough for a second interaction that anchors the platelet to the damaged site. This firm adhesion can be mediated by several membrane receptors, some of which will have become activated as a result of platelet rolling and others who are expressed on the platelet surface as a result platelet activation (Jackson et al., 2009). Once firmly adhered, the platelets rearrange cytoskeletal components which results in filopodia and llamelipodia extension leading to flattening or spreading of the platelet. Platelet spreading is critical following firm adhesion as it firstly allows the platelet withstand the shear forces experienced in the vasculature and secondly it increases the platelet surface area thus covering more of the damaged site.

Following attachment, platelets undergo a series of highly controlled intracellular signalling events that lead to the release reaction where platelets release the contents of its stored intracellular granules. Alpha granules contain proteins such as P-selectin which mediates adhesion of platelets to monocytes, neutrophils and lymphocytes, resulting in the formation of platelet leukocyte complexes (Diacovo et al., 1996a, Diacovo et al., 1996b, Larsen et al., 1989). These granules also contain many chemotactic agents which lead to the recruitment of various inflammatory cells; platelet derived growth factor (PDGF) and 12-hydroxyeicosate-traenoic acid (12-HETE) which recruit neutrophils (Herd and Page, 1994, Mannaioni et al., 1997); platelet factor 4 and platelet derived histamine releasing factor (PDHRF) which recruit eosinophils in airway disease (Brindley et al., 1983, Frigas and Gleich, 1986); PDGF and transforming growth factor β (TGF-β) which recruit monocytes and macrophages and TGF-β which recruits fibroblasts (Deuel et al., 1982, Tzeng et al., 1985, Wahl et al., 1987). Platelet granules also contain several mediators of tissue damage such as oxygen free radicals and hydrolytic enzymes. Dense granules release cationic proteins that initiate vascular permeability and mediators that enhance aggregate formation such as adenosine diphosphate (ADP) and serotonin (5-HT) (Rendu and Brohard-Bohn, 2001). Bioactive amines are also secreted from platelets following activation including Thromboxane A_2 (TxA2) and platelet activating factor (PAF) (McIntyre et al., 2003, Patrono et al., 2001).More recently it has been shown that platelet granules contain many antimicrobial peptides such as beta-lysin, platelet microbial protein (PMP), neutrophil activating peptide (NAP-2), released upon activation normal T-cell expressed and secreted (RANTES) and fibrinopeptides A and B (Johnson and Donaldson, 1968, Donaldson and Tew, 1977, Kameyoshi et al., 1992, Yeaman et al., 1997, Krijgsveld et al., 2000).

Once activation is complete the platelet forms a new surface for additional platelets to adhere, predominantly through GPIIb/IIIa crosslinking adjacent platelets through a fibrinogen bridge, resulting in aggregate formation. The final step sees and effective plug at the site of injury that is reinforced by the conversion of fibrinogen to fibrin through the coagulation cascade (Ruggeri et al., 2006).

4. The growing role of platelets in infection and immunity

Platelets are poorly recognised for their role in infection and immunity even though just like professional phagocytes (neutrophils, macrophages and dendritic cells) platelets are derived from the same haematopoietic stem cell, undergo chemotaxis (Clemetson et al., 2000), phagocytose foreign particles (Youssefian et al., 2002), and secrete a multitude of products including inflammatory mediators (Kameyoshi et al., 1992), cytokines (Lindemann et al., 2001a, Antczak et al., 2010) and antimicrobial peptides (Tang et al., 2002, Mercier et al., 2004), all while directing and recruiting several members of the innate immune system to the infected area (Cox et al., 2011, Semple and Freedman, 2010). In addition, toll like receptors (TLR) which are a family of pattern recognition receptors expressed by several professional phagocytes recognise conserved molecular motifs expressed on different classes of infectious agent (Janeway and Medzhitov, 2002, Armant and Fenton, 2002). To date at least 13 TLRs have been described in various immune and nonimmune cells in both human and mice. Recently human platelet have been shown to express TLR1,2,4,6,8 and 9, reinforcing their role as primitive immune cells in host defence (Cognasse et al., 2005, Shiraki et al., 2004, Aslam et al., 2006, Zhang et al., 2009, Garraud and Cognasse, 2010, Andonegui et al., 2005, Keane et al., 2010). More recent studies have also demonstrated that TLRs are also responsible for lipopolysaccharide (LPS)-induced thrombocytopenia (Andonegui et al., 2005, Aslam et al., 2006).

5. Mechanisms of interaction

Bacteria can interact with platelet in two ways, they can either support platelet adhesion or they can induce platelet aggregation. Platelet adhesion to immobilised bacteria is a measure of the strength of the interaction, whereas platelet aggregation induced by bacteria is a measure of the quality of the interaction. In contrast to typical platelet aggregation induced by physiological agonists such as adenosine diphosphate (ADP), collagen or thrombin, bacteria induce an all or nothing response. This means that the bacteria either induce a maximal aggregation or they don't induce platelet aggregation at all, there is no intermediate response. Another unique feature of bacteria induced platelet aggregation is a distinct pause in time before aggregation takes place. This is typically called the lag time. Increasing the concentration of bacteria shortens the lag time but never eliminates it. The average lag time to platelet aggregation following addition of Staphylococci is between 5-12 minutes. This is in contrast to the lag time observed upon the addition of typical platelet agonists ADP or thrombin which have a lag time less than 10 seconds.

There are 3 main interactions between bacteria and platelets. In the first interaction bacteria express proteins that can directly interact with a surface receptor on the platelet. In this case the bacterial protein express ligand mimetic domains that act as agonists on the platelet receptor thus triggering an intracellular signal that culminates in platelet activation. In the second interaction bacterial proteins bind a plasma protein that is a natural ligand for a platelet receptor. For example, bacteria can bind antibody which in turn bridges the bacteria to the antibody receptor (FcγRIIa) expressed on the platelet. Once engaged the receptor results in the generation of an intracellular signal leading to platelet activation. Finally bacteria may have the ability to secrete products or toxins that in turn activate platelets. Engagement of the product or toxin with a platelet receptor results in activation. These different mechanisms of interaction may help explain the lag time to platelet aggregation. For example, the lag time could be representative of the time taken to trigger a response or bind a plasma protein. A major challenge in studying platelet bacterial interactions is that most bacteria can interact with platelets using multiple mechanisms. This makes it incredibly difficult to identify either the platelet receptors or the bacterial proteins involved in triggering thrombus formation. Moreover not only are the interactions species specific but strain specific as well.

6. Staphylococci interactions with platelets

6.1. Indirect interaction (Released products)

Staphylococcus aureus was one of the first bacteria isolated from patients with acute endocarditis. Despite improvements in medical and surgical therapy, invasive staphylococcal disease causing infective endocarditis is still the most frequent etiologic microorganism found in patients (Rasmussen et al., 2011). Studies investigating the mechanism through which *S. aureus* contributes to endocarditis dates back as far as the early 1900's. By the mid 1900's significant attention had been placed on the involvement of *S. aureus* alpha (α)-toxin in contributing to IE. Alpha-toxin is produced by almost all strains of *S. aureus*. Typically α-toxin disrupts the cell membrane by binding to the lipid bilayer of platelets, erythrocytes and some leukocytes, forming an oligomeric structure that forms a water filled transmembrane pore. In 1964 Siegel and Cohen made two critical observations; first, addition of α-toxin led to the loss of single platelets as evidenced by turbidimetric aggregometry and second that addition of α-toxin to human platelets resulted in leakage of intracellular ions; NAD+, K+ and ATP but interestingly not protein, suggesting that α-toxin was not lysing the platelets (Siegel and Cohen, 1964). Further studies by Bernheimer and Schwartz confirmed these reports and demonstrated by electron microscopy that following exposure to α-toxin platelets swelled but did not show signs of lysis (Bernheimer, 1965). These early studies suggested that α-toxin may have the ability to generate a signal upon binding to the platelet. Focusing on this Arvand and colleagues demonstrated that α-toxin did indeed trigger a platelet signal upon binding and most importantly one that leads to secretion of intracellular contents including procoagulant mediators, platelet factor 4 and factor V. Secreted factor V in turn associates with the platelet membrane leading to assembly of the prothrombinase complex (Arvand et al., 1990). This explains the major pathway responsible for the procoagulatory effects of α-toxin. In contrast to these early findings Bayer et al. demonstrated that α-toxin did cause platelet lysis and this led to the release of platelet microbial proteins (PMP's) which was bactericidal to *S. aureus*.

Using an animal model of endocarditis the authors demonstrated that different strains of *S. aureus* differed in the expression of functional versus mutant forms of α-toxin. Under these conditions, the *S. aureus* strains producing either minimal or no α-toxin were less virulent *in vivo* than wild-type strains (Bayer et al., 1997). Wild-type *S. aureus* strains or indeed an isogenic strain engineered to over-express α-toxin were associated with increased release of PMP from platelets. These results suggest that when *S. aureus* releases α-toxin, platelets release PMP's therefore leading to a protective role for the host by destroying *S. aureus*.

Lipoteichoic acid (LTA) is an essential component of the cell wall of *S. aureus* and plays a key role in host-pathogen interactions (Morath et al., 2005). LTA is anchored to the cell wall via diacylglycerol, however following bacteriolysis induced by cationic proteins from leukocytes or antibiotic treatment with certain antibiotics, LTA is released from the cell wall (Lotz et al., 2006). LTA is a very potent stimulator of cells expressing the pattern recognition receptor, toll like receptor 2 (TLR2) (Kawai and Akira, 2010). Functional TLR2 is expressed on a number of immune cells including platelets (Blair et al., 2009, Keane et al., 2010, Ward et al., 2005). Work by Sheu et al, demonstrated that LTA from *S. aureus* inhibited platelet aggregation, calcium mobilisation and cyclic AMP in human platelets (Sheu et al., 2000a, Sheu et al., 2000b). It remains to be seen whether TLR2 is mediating this inhibition of platelet signalling.

6.2. Indirect interaction (Cell wall proteins)

There are numerous cell wall proteins expressed on the surface of *S. aureus* that have been demonstrated to bind to platelets and trigger platelet activation. The majority of these cell wall proteins have been found to bind plasma proteins and bridge to a platelet receptor. Staphylococcal protein A is a widely expressed protein found on greater than 90% of *S. aureus* strains. In 1979, Hawiger et al., demonstrated that protein A is capable of binding to immunoglobulin G (IgG) which in turn bridges to the platelet antibody receptor, FcγRIIa. This interaction results in platelet signal generation, GPIIbIIIa dependent platelet aggregation and serotonin release from the platelet dense granules. Interestingly purified protein A failed to cause measureable platelet aggregation and release of serotonin was significantly reduced (Hawiger et al., 1979). Recent studies have demonstrated that protein A can bind to the A1 domain of the major plasma protein vonWillebrand factor with high affinity (low nM range) (O'Seaghdha et al., 2006) which serves as a receptor for GPIbα expressed on platelets (Andrews et al., 2003). More recent studies have investigated this interaction under fluid shear conditions and demonstrated that preincubating platelet rich plasma with a vonWillebrand Factor antibody or indeed blocking the platelet GPIbα receptor with an inhibitory monoclonal antibody partially inhibited the platelet-*S. aureus* interaction. Furthermore using a strain of *S. aureus* that is deficient in protein A expression reduced its interactions with platelets (Pawar et al., 2004).These results suggest that protein A plays a role in triggering platelet activation.

More recent studies demonstrated that multiple cell wall proteins expressed on *S. aureus* are capable of interacting with and triggering platelet aggregation (O'Brien et al., 2002). Among the cell wall proteins identified, clumping factor A (ClfA) and clumping factor B (ClfB) are possibly the most extensively studied. ClfA and ClfB has been shown to bind a number of plasma proteins including fibrinogen, IgG and complement, which in turn bridge the bacteria to specific platelet receptors and trigger activation. Binding each plasma protein individually is not sufficient to trigger platelet aggregation. To trigger full platelet activation ClfA or ClfB must bind specific IgG along with either fibrinogen or complement, IgG being the key molecule. There are at least two distinct sites on each ClfA or ClfB that allows IgG and fibrinogen bind at the same time. Once this occurs, fibrinogen binds to platelet GPIIbIIIa, IgG binds to platelet FcγRIIa and together induces receptor clustering leading to activation of signal transduction pathways culminating in platelet aggregation (Loughman et al., 2005, Miajlovic et al., 2007). Deletion of the fibrinogen binding domain on ClfA or ClfB led to the discovery of another much slower platelet aggregation (8-20 minutes versus 2-4 minutes). Loughman et al initially demonstrated that complement must assemble on the *S. aureus* surface and then cross link to complement receptors expressed on platelets. Similar to before, IgG binds to FcγRIIa, complement proteins binds to complement receptors on platelets and together induces receptor clustering leading to activation of signal transduction pathways culminating in platelet aggregation (Loughman et al., 2005). Much controversy surrounds the existence of complement receptors on platelets however the most convincing evidence of a complement receptor is that demonstrated by Nyugen et al., who demonstrated the expression of gC1qR/p33 following platelet activation. This suggests that an initial interaction leads to platelet activation which in turn triggers expression of gC1qR/p33 on the platelet surface. Expression of this receptor post activation most likely serves to anchor the bacteria to the platelet.

A critical part of *S. aureus* survival in the host is the wide array of cell wall proteins it expresses at various growth phases of its cell cycle. For example, ClfA is weakly expressed during the exponential phase and strongly expressed during the stationary phase. In contrast to this fibronectin binding protein A (FnbpA) is strongly expressed during the exponential phase of growth and weakly expressed during the stationary phase of growth. FnbpA also plays a key role in inducing platelet aggregation. The mechanism through which FnbpA induces platelet aggregation is more or less identical to the mechanism that ClfA uses to induce platelet aggregation. Fnbp contain a specific immunoglobulin binding domain (A domain) and a separate fibronectin binding domain (BCD). FnBPA possesses two different but related mechanisms of engaging and activating platelets (Fitzgerald et al., 2006). In the first mechanism, fibrinogen can bind to the A domain which crosslinks to GPIIb/IIIa, and specific immunoglobulin must crosslink to FcγRIIa to trigger platelet activation and aggregation (Fitzgerald et al., 2006). In the second mechanism fibronectin can bind to *S. aureus* via the FnBPA BCD domain (Meenan et al., 2007, Raibaud et al., 2005). The signal to trigger platelet activation/aggregation is complete when specific immunoglobulin binds the A domain of FnBPA and cross links to platelet FcγRIIa inducing receptor clustering.

As discussed in chapter 2 serine rich proteins expressed by viridans streptococci play a critical role in inducing platelet aggregation. *S. aureus* also expresses a highly glycosylated serine rich protein called SraP on its surface (Siboo et al., 2005). Strain of *S. aureus* deficient in expression of SraP has been shown to have reduced virulence in a rabbit model of endocarditis. Regardless of the fact that SraP shares significant similarities with a number of other serine rich glycoproteins found in the streptococci that have been found to bind to platelet GPIbα (Kerrigan et al., 2007, Plummer et al., 2005), SraP does not appear to bind to this platelet receptor.

While all of these studies are critical to our understanding of the molecular mechanisms involved in aggregate formation, one must be aware of the relevance of these findings to physiological conditions experienced in the vasculature. For example, almost all of the studies carried out to date have been carried out under non-physiological stirring or using static adhesion assays, neither of which are representative of the conditions experienced in the vasculature. Many reports in the literature in recent times have clearly demonstrated that the local fluid environment in the circulation critically affects the molecular pathways of cell-cell interactions (Varki, 1994). To address this several attempts have been made to create an environment more representative of conditions experienced in the circulation. Rheology is a useful technique that can be employed to shear cells at physiological rates. Using a cone and plate viscometer, Pawar et al. demonstrated that when *S. aureus* is mixed with whole blood isolated from a healthy individual thrombus formation could be observed. Additional studies demonstrated that the thrombus formation was dependent on multiple *S. aureus* cell wall proteins including protein A, ClfA, SdrC, SdrD, SdrE (Pawar et al., 2004). A potential limitation to using a cone and plate viscometer is that is measures thrombus formation in a soluble setting and it is well established that thrombus formation on a heart valve in IE occurs under stable conditions. To address this Kerrigan et al. developed a parallel flow chamber to assess the interaction between *S. aureus* and platelets in whole blood. To do this *S. aureus* was immobilised on a glass slide (to mimic the focal infection on a heart valve) and whole blood was perfused over the bacteria at both arterial and venous shear rates. This method demonstrated that platelets perfused over immobilised *S. aureus* under arterial shear led to a very strong adhesion, followed by rapid aggregate formation. Deletion of ClfA (but not protein A or FnbpA) from *S. aureus* abolished adhesion and subsequent aggregate formation. Using a plasma-free system, fibrinogen led to single platelet adhesion but not aggregate formation. Specific immunoglobulin failed to have any effect on either platelet adhesion or aggregation. However, addition of fibrinogen and specific immunoglobulin together to the plasma-free system led to platelet adhesion followed by aggregate formation thus highlighting the importance of fibrinogen and IgG in aggregate formation. Interestingly platelets did not adhere to or induce aggregate formation under low shear conditions using the parallel flow chamber (Kerrigan et al., 2008).

6.3. Direct interaction (Cell wall proteins)

A growing concern about studies to date is the apparent lack of contrast with conditions experienced physiologically. *In vivo,* when *S. aureus* enters the blood stream it is in an environment where iron is sequestered in haem or haemoglobulin. The lack of iron available *in vivo* inactivates the Fur repressor in *S. aureus* that results in an up-regulation of a number of genes that typically wouldn't be expressed in when growing in normal laboratory bacterial growth media. A growing family of iron-regulated surface determinant proteins have been recently identified as expressed in *S. aureus* grown in iron limited conditions. Using surface plasmon resonance, Miajlovic et al. demonstrated that one family member, iron-regulated surface determinant B (IsdB), can bind directly (in the absence of plasma proteins) to the purified platelet fibrinogen receptor GPIIb/IIIa. As a result of this binding subsequent studies demonstrated the ability of the wildtype *S. aureus* strain to support platelet adhesion and induce platelet aggregation. A. *S. aureus* strain defective in expression of IsdB displayed a reduce ability to adhere to or induce platelet aggregation (Miajlovic et al., 2010).

7. Final thoughts and future directions

Infective endocarditis is notoriously difficult to treat as antibiotics are incapable of penetrating the growing thrombus to reach the encased microorganisms. As a result of this the in-hospital mortality rate can be as high as 36% (Botelho-Nevers et al., 2009). Even with treatment, 40% of patients with infective endocarditis relapse within 2 months of finishing clinically effective therapy (Netzer et al., 2002). Furthermore, approximately 25% of patients with infective endocarditis eventually require surgery, usually within 2 years after completing therapy (Olaison and Pettersson, 2003). These statistics reflect the poor delivery and penetration of antibiotic into the growing thrombus. The costs associated with hospitalization (of which the average stay in hospital is 30 days), surgery and prolonged antibiotic treatment is extremely high placing a severe burden on already over-stretched healthcare systems though out the world. The danger of *S. aureus* invasive disease is also compounded by the rapidly increasing global widespread occurrence of multiple antibiotic resistant strains (MRSA and VRSA) which is directly attributed to prolong use of antibiotics. The greater the duration of exposure of an antibiotic to bacteria, the greater the risk of development of resistance and this is irrespective of the severity of the need for antibiotics. If this is not addressed soon, acquired resistance may produce a virtually untreatable pathogen. Therefore it is of the utmost importance that we understand the molecular interactions that lead to the development of thrombus formation on the heart valves. This will serve two purposes, first it may lead to the development of novel therapies that will prevent the formation of a thrombus on the heart valve and secondly as a result will overcome the problem associated with getting clinically effective concentrations of antibiotic to the site of infection on the heart valve.

Potential drug targets identified from studies over the years suggest that blocking the interaction between IgG and platelet FcγRIIa may indeed prevent platelet receptor clustering and thus inhibit thrombus formation. Blockade of the platelet FcγRIIa receptor has distinct advantages over other anti-platelet agents as inhibitors of FcγRIIa do not affect the platelet response to other agonist and therefore does not compromise essential platelet functions.

Author details

Steven W. Kerrigan

School of Pharmacy & Molecular and Cellular Therapeutics, Royal College of Surgeons in Ireland, Dublin, Ireland

References

[1] Andonegui, G, Kerfoot, S. M, Mcnagny, K, Ebbert, K. V, Patel, K. D, & Kubes, P. (2005). Platelets express functional Toll-like receptor-4. *Blood*, , 106, 2417-23.

[2] Andrews, R. K, Gardiner, E. E, Shen, Y, & Berndt, M. C. (2003). Structure-activity relationships of snake toxins targeting platelet receptors, glycoprotein Ib-IX-V and glycoprotein VI. *Curr Med Chem Cardiovasc Hematol Agents*, , 1, 143-9.

[3] Antczak, A. J, Singh, N, Gay, S. R, & Worth, R. G. (2010). IgG-complex stimulated platelets: a source of sCD40L and RANTES in initiation of inflammatory cascade. *Cell Immunol*, , 263, 129-33.

[4] Armant, M. A, & Fenton, M. J. (2002). Toll-like receptors: a family of pattern-recognition receptors in mammals. *Genome Biol*, 3, REVIEWS3011.

[5] Arvand, M, Bhakdi, S, Dahlback, B, & Preissner, K. T. (1990). Staphylococcus aureus alpha-toxin attack on human platelets promotes assembly of the prothrombinase complex. *J Biol Chem*, , 265, 14377-81.

[6] Aslam, R, Speck, E. R, Kim, M, Crow, A. R, Bang, K. W, Nestel, F. P, Ni, H, Lazarus, A. H, Freedman, J, & Semple, J. W. (2006). Platelet Toll-like receptor expression modulates lipopolysaccharide-induced thrombocytopenia and tumor necrosis factor-alpha production in vivo. *Blood*, , 107, 637-41.

[7] Bayer, A. S, Ramos, M. D, Menzies, B. E, Yeaman, M. R, Shen, A. J, & Cheung, A. L. (1997). Hyperproduction of alpha-toxin by Staphylococcus aureus results in paradoxically reduced virulence in experimental endocarditis: a host defense role for platelet microbicidal proteins. *Infect Immun*, , 65, 4652-60.

[8] Bernheimer, A. W. (1965). Staphylococcal alpha toxin. *Ann N Y Acad Sci*, , 128, 112-23.

[9] Blair, P, Rex, S, Vitseva, O, Beaulieu, L, Tanriverdi, K, Chakrabarti, S, Hayashi, C, Genco, C. A, Iafrati, M, & Freedman, J. E. (2009). Stimulation of Toll-like receptor 2 in human platelets induces a thromboinflammatory response through activation of phosphoinositide 3-kinase. *Circ Res*, , 104, 346-54.

[10] Botelho-nevers, E, Thuny, F, Casalta, J. P, Richet, H, Gouriet, F, Collart, F, Riberi, A, Habib, G, & Raoult, D. (2009). Dramatic reduction in infective endocarditis-related mortality with a management-based approach. *Arch Intern Med*, , 169, 1290-8.

[11] Brindley, L. L, Sweet, J. M, & Goetzl, E. J. (1983). Stimulation of histamine release from human basophils by human platelet factor 4. *J Clin Invest*, , 72, 1218-23.

[12] Castillo, J. C, Anguita, M. P, Ramirez, A, Siles, J. R, Torres, F, Mesa, D, Franco, M, Munoz, I, Concha, M, & Valles, F. (2000). Long term outcome of infective endocarditis in patients who were not drug addicts: a 10 year study. *Heart*, , 83, 525-30.

[13] Chesterman, C. N, & Berndt, M. C. (1986). Platelet and vessel wall interaction and the genesis of atherosclerosis. *Clin Haematol*, , 15, 323-53.

[14] Clemetson, K. J, Clemetson, J. M, Proudfoot, A. E, Power, C. A, Baggiolini, M, & Wells, T. N. (2000). Functional expression of CCR1, CCR3, CCR4, and CXCR4 chemokine receptors on human platelets. *Blood*, , 96, 4046-54.

[15] Cognasse, F, Hamzeh, H, Chavarin, P, Acquart, S, Genin, C, & Garraud, O. (2005). Evidence of Toll-like receptor molecules on human platelets. *Immunol Cell Biol*, , 83, 196-8.

[16] Cox, D, Kerrigan, S. W, & Watson, S. P. (2011). Platelets and the innate immune system: mechanisms of bacterial-induced platelet activation. *J Thromb Haemost*, , 9, 1097-107.

[17] Deuel, T. F, Senior, R. M, Huang, J. S, & Griffin, G. L. (1982). Chemotaxis of monocytes and neutrophils to platelet-derived growth factor. *J Clin Invest*, , 69, 1046-9.

[18] Diacovo, T. G, Puri, K. D, Warnock, R. A, Springer, T. A, & Von Andrian, U. H. lymphocyte delivery to high endothelial venules. *Science*, , 273, 252-5.

[19] Diacovo, T. G, Roth, S. J, Buccola, J. M, Bainton, D. F, & Springer, T. A. (1996b). Neutrophil rolling, arrest, and transmigration across activated, surface-adherent platelets via sequential action of P-selectin and the beta 2-integrin CD11b/CD18. *Blood*, , 88, 146-57.

[20] Donaldson, D. M, & Tew, J. G. (1977). beta-Lysin of platelet origin. *Bacteriol Rev*, , 41, 501-13.

[21] Durack, D. T. (1995). Prevention of infective endocarditis. *N Engl J Med*, , 332, 38-44.

[22] Fitzgerald, J. R, Loughman, A, Keane, F, Brennan, M, Knobel, M, Higgins, J, Visai, L, Speziale, P, Cox, D, & Foster, T. J. (2006). Fibronectin-binding proteins of Staphylococcus aureus mediate activation of human platelets via fibrinogen and fibronectin bridges to integrin GPIIb/IIIa and IgG binding to the FcgammaRIIa receptor. *Mol Microbiol*, , 59, 212-30.

[23] Foster, T. J. (2009). Colonization and infection of the human host by staphylococci: adhesion, survival and immune evasion. *Vet Dermatol*, , 20, 456-70.

[24] Frigas, E, & Gleich, G. J. (1986). The eosinophil and the pathophysiology of asthma. *J Allergy Clin Immunol*, , 77, 527-37.

[25] Garraud, O, & Cognasse, F. (2010). Platelet Toll-like receptor expression: the link between "danger" ligands and inflammation. *Inflamm Allergy Drug Targets*, , 9, 322-33.

[26] Gawaz, M, Langer, H, & May, A. E. (2005). Platelets in inflammation and atherogenesis. *J Clin Invest*, , 115, 3378-84.

[27] George, N. P, Wei, Q, Shin, P. K, Konstantopoulos, K, & Ross, J. M. (2006). Staphylococcus aureus adhesion via Spa, ClfA, and SdrCDE to immobilized platelets demonstrates shear-dependent behavior. *Arterioscler Thromb Vasc Biol*, , 26, 2394-400.

[28] Hawiger, J, Steckley, S, Hammond, D, Cheng, C, Timmons, S, & Glick, A. D. Des Prez, R. M. (1979). Staphylococci-induced human platelet injury mediated by protein A and immunoglobulin G Fc fragment receptor. *J Clin Invest*, , 64, 931-7.

[29] Heiro, M, Nikoskelainen, J, Engblom, E, Kotilainen, E, Marttila, R, & Kotilainen, P. (2000). Neurologic manifestations of infective endocarditis: a 17-year experience in a teaching hospital in Finland. *Arch Intern Med*, , 160, 2781-7.

[30] Herd, C. M, & Page, C. P. (1994). Pulmonary immune cells in health and disease: platelets. *Eur Respir J*, , 7, 1145-60.

[31] Jackson, S. P, Nesbitt, W. S, & Westein, E. (2009). Dynamics of platelet thrombus formation. *J Thromb Haemost,* 7 Suppl , 1, 17-20.

[32] Janeway, C. A. Jr. & Medzhitov, R. (2002). Innate immune recognition. *Annu Rev Immunol*, , 20, 197-216.

[33] Jault, F, Gandjbakhch, I, Rama, A, Nectoux, M, Bors, V, Vaissier, E, Nataf, P, Pavie, A, & Cabrol, C. (1997). Active native valve endocarditis: determinants of operative death and late mortality. *Ann Thorac Surg*, , 63, 1737-41.

[34] Johnson, F. B, & Donaldson, D. M. (1968). Purification of staphylocidal beta-lysin from rabbit serum. *J Bacteriol*, , 96, 589-95.

[35] Jurk, K, Clemetson, K. J, De Groot, P. G, Brodde, M. F, Steiner, M, Savion, N, Varon, D, Sixma, J. J, Van Aken, H, & Kehrel, B. E. (2003). Thrombospondin-1 mediates platelet adhesion at high shear via glycoprotein Ib (GPIb): an alternative/backup mechanism to von Willebrand factor. *FASEB J*, , 17, 1490-2.

[36] Kameyoshi, Y, Dorschner, A, Mallet, A. I, Christophers, E, & Schroder, J. M. (1992). Cytokine RANTES released by thrombin-stimulated platelets is a potent attractant for human eosinophils. *J Exp Med*, , 176, 587-92.

[37] Kasirer-friede, A, Kahn, M. L, & Shattil, S. J. (2007). Platelet integrins and immunoreceptors. *Immunol Rev*, , 218, 247-64.

[38] Kawai, T, & Akira, S. (2010). The role of pattern-recognition receptors in innate immunity: update on Toll-like receptors. *Nat Immunol*, , 11, 373-84.

[39] Keane, C, Tilley, D, Cunningham, A, Smolenski, A, Kadioglu, A, Cox, D, Jenkinson, H. F, & Kerrigan, S. W. (2010). Invasive Streptococcus pneumoniae trigger platelet activation via Toll-like receptor 2. *J Thromb Haemost*, , 8, 2757-65.

[40] Kerrigan, S. W, Clarke, N, Loughman, A, Meade, G, Foster, T. J, & Cox, D. (2008). Molecular basis for Staphylococcus aureus-mediated platelet aggregate formation under arterial shear in vitro. *Arterioscler Thromb Vasc Biol*, , 28, 335-40.

[41] Kerrigan, S. W, Jakubovics, N. S, Keane, C, Maguire, P, Wynne, K, Jenkinson, H. F, & Cox, D. (2007). Role of Streptococcus gordonii surface proteins SspA/SspB and Hsa in platelet function. *Infect Immun,* , 75, 5740-7.

[42] Krijgsveld, J, Zaat, S. A, Meeldijk, J, Van Veelen, P. A, Fang, G, Poolman, B, Brandt, E, Ehlert, J. E, Kuijpers, A. J, Engbers, G. H, Feijen, J, & Dankert, J. (2000). Thrombocidins, microbicidal proteins from human blood platelets, are C-terminal deletion products of CXC chemokines. *J Biol Chem,* , 275, 20374-81.

[43] Larsen, E, Celi, A, Gilbert, G. E, Furie, B. C, Erban, J. K, Bonfanti, R, Wagner, D. D, & Furie, B. (1989). Padgem protein: a receptor that mediates the interaction of activated platelets with neutrophils and monocytes. *Cell,* , 59, 305-12.

[44] Lindemann, S, Tolley, N. D, Dixon, D. A, Mcintyre, T. M, Prescott, S. M, Zimmerman, G. A, & Weyrich, A. S. (2001a). Activated platelets mediate inflammatory signaling by regulated interleukin 1beta synthesis. *J Cell Biol,* , 154, 485-90.

[45] Lindemann, S, Tolley, N. D, Eyre, J. R, Kraiss, L. W, Mahoney, T. M, & Weyrich, A. S. (2001b). Integrins regulate the intracellular distribution of eukaryotic initiation factor 4E in platelets. A checkpoint for translational control. *J Biol Chem,* , 276, 33947-51.

[46] Lotz, S, Starke, A, Ziemann, C, Morath, S, Hartung, T, Solbach, W, & Laskay, T. (2006). Beta-lactam antibiotic-induced release of lipoteichoic acid from Staphylococcus aureus leads to activation of neutrophil granulocytes. *Ann Clin Microbiol Antimicrob,* 5, 15.

[47] Loughman, A, Fitzgerald, J. R, Brennan, M. P, Higgins, J, Downer, R, Cox, D, & Foster, T. J. (2005). Roles for fibrinogen, immunoglobulin and complement in platelet activation promoted by Staphylococcus aureus clumping factor A. *Mol Microbiol,* , 57, 804-18.

[48] Mannaioni, P. F. Di Bello, M. G. & Masini, E. (1997). Platelets and inflammation: role of platelet-derived growth factor, adhesion molecules and histamine. *Inflamm Res,* , 46, 4-18.

[49] Mcintyre, T. M, Prescott, S. M, Weyrich, A. S, & Zimmerman, G. A. (2003). Cell-cell interactions: leukocyte-endothelial interactions. *Curr Opin Hematol,* , 10, 150-8.

[50] Meenan, N. A, Visai, L, Valtulina, V, Schwarz-linek, U, Norris, N. C, Gurusiddappa, S, Hook, M, Speziale, P, & Potts, J. R. (2007). The tandem beta-zipper model defines high affinity fibronectin-binding repeats within Staphylococcus aureus FnBPA. *J Biol Chem,* , 282, 25893-902.

[51] Mercier, R. C, Dietz, R. M, Mazzola, J. L, Bayer, A. S, & Yeaman, M. R. (2004). Beneficial influence of platelets on antibiotic efficacy in an in vitro model of Staphylococcus aureus-induced endocarditis. *Antimicrob Agents Chemother,* , 48, 2551-7.

[52] Miajlovic, H, Loughman, A, Brennan, M, Cox, D, & Foster, T. J. (2007). Both complement- and fibrinogen-dependent mechanisms contribute to platelet aggregation mediated by Staphylococcus aureus clumping factor B. *Infect Immun,* , 75, 3335-43.

[53] Miajlovic, H, Zapotoczna, M, Geoghegan, J. A, Kerrigan, S. W, Speziale, P, & Foster, T. J. (2010). Direct interaction of iron-regulated surface determinant IsdB of Staphylococcus aureus with the GPIIb/IIIa receptor on platelets. *Microbiology,* , 156, 920-8.

[54] Morath, S, Von Aulock, S, & Hartung, T. (2005). Structure/function relationships of lipoteichoic acids. *J Endotoxin Res,* , 11, 348-56.

[55] Moreillon, P, & Que, Y. A. (2004). Infective endocarditis. *Lancet,* , 363, 139-49.

[56] Murdoch, D. R, Corey, G. R, Hoen, B, Miro, J. M, & Fowler, V. G. Jr., Bayer, A. S., Karchmer, A. W., Olaison, L., Pappas, P. A., Moreillon, P., Chambers, S. T., Chu, V. H., Falco, V., Holland, D. J., Jones, P., Klein, J. L., Raymond, N. J., Read, K. M., Tripodi, M. F., Utili, R., Wang, A., Woods, C. W. & Cabell, C. H. (2009). Clinical presentation, etiology, and outcome of infective endocarditis in the 21st century: the International Collaboration on Endocarditis-Prospective Cohort Study. *Arch Intern Med,* , 169, 463-73.

[57] Netzer, R. O, Altwegg, S. C, Zollinger, E, Tauber, M, Carrel, T, & Seiler, C. (2002). Infective endocarditis: determinants of long term outcome. *Heart,* , 88, 61-6.

[58] Nieswandt, B, Varga-szabo, D, & Elvers, M. (2009). Integrins in platelet activation. *J Thromb Haemost,* 7 Suppl , 1, 206-9.

[59] Brien, O, Kerrigan, L, Kaw, S. W, Hogan, G, Penades, M, Litt, J, Fitzgerald, D, Foster, D. J, & Cox, T. J. D. (2002). Multiple mechanisms for the activation of human platelet aggregation by Staphylococcus aureus: roles for the clumping factors ClfA and ClfB, the serine-aspartate repeat protein SdrE and protein A. *Mol Microbiol,* , 44, 1033-44.

[60] Seaghdha, O, Van Schooten, M, Kerrigan, C. J, Emsley, S. W, Silverman, J, Cox, G. J, Lenting, D, & Foster, P. J. T. J. (2006). Staphylococcus aureus protein A binding to von Willebrand factor A1 domain is mediated by conserved IgG binding regions. *FEBS J,* , 273, 4831-41.

[61] Olaison, L, & Pettersson, G. (2003). Current best practices and guidelines. Indications for surgical intervention in infective endocarditis. *Cardiol Clin,* vii., 21, 235-51.

[62] Patrono, C, & Patrignani, P. Garcia Rodriguez, L. A. (2001). Cyclooxygenase-selective inhibition of prostanoid formation: transducing biochemical selectivity into clinical read-outs. *J Clin Invest,* , 108, 7-13.

[63] Patti, J. M, Allen, B. L, Mcgavin, M. J, & Hook, M. (1994). MSCRAMM-mediated adherence of microorganisms to host tissues. *Annu Rev Microbiol,* , 48, 585-617.

[64] Pawar, P, Shin, P. K, Mousa, S. A, Ross, J. M, & Konstantopoulos, K. (2004). Fluid shear regulates the kinetics and receptor specificity of Staphylococcus aureus binding to activated platelets. *J Immunol*, , 173, 1258-65.

[65] Plummer, C, Wu, H, Kerrigan, S. W, Meade, G, & Cox, D. Ian Douglas, C. W. (2005). A serine-rich glycoprotein of Streptococcus sanguis mediates adhesion to platelets via GPIb. *Br J Haematol*, , 129, 101-9.

[66] Prendergast, B. D, & Tornos, P. (2010). Surgery for infective endocarditis: who and when? *Circulation*, , 121, 1141-52.

[67] Raibaud, S, Schwarz-linek, U, Kim, J. H, Jenkins, H. T, Baines, E. R, Gurusiddappa, S, Hook, M, & Potts, J. R. (2005). Borrelia burgdorferi binds fibronectin through a tandem beta-zipper, a common mechanism of fibronectin binding in staphylococci, streptococci, and spirochetes. *J Biol Chem*, , 280, 18803-9.

[68] Rasmussen, R. V, Host, U, Arpi, M, Hassager, C, Johansen, H. K, Korup, E, Schonheyder, H. C, Berning, J, Gill, S, Rosenvinge, F. S, & Fowler, V. G. Jr., Moller, J. E., Skov, R. L., Larsen, C. T., Hansen, T. F., Mard, S., Smit, J., Andersen, P. S. & Bruun, N. E. (2011). Prevalence of infective endocarditis in patients with Staphylococcus aureus bacteraemia: the value of screening with echocardiography. *Eur J Echocardiogr*, , 12, 414-20.

[69] Remadi, J. P, Habib, G, Nadji, G, Brahim, A, Thuny, F, Casalta, J. P, Peltier, M, & Tribouilloy, C. (2007). Predictors of death and impact of surgery in Staphylococcus aureus infective endocarditis. *Ann Thorac Surg*, , 83, 1295-302.

[70] Rendu, F, & Brohard-bohn, B. (2001). The platelet release reaction: granules' constituents, secretion and functions. *Platelets*, , 12, 261-73.

[71] Ruggeri, Z. M. (1999). Structure and function of von Willebrand factor. *Thromb Haemost*, , 82, 576-84.

[72] Ruggeri, Z. M. (2009). Platelet adhesion under flow. *Microcirculation*, , 16, 58-83.

[73] Ruggeri, Z. M, & Mendolicchio, G. L. (2007). Adhesion mechanisms in platelet function. *Circ Res*, , 100, 1673-85.

[74] Ruggeri, Z. M, Orje, J. N, Habermann, R, Federici, A. B, & Reininger, A. J. (2006). Activation-independent platelet adhesion and aggregation under elevated shear stress. *Blood*, , 108, 1903-10.

[75] Santoro, S. A, & Zutter, M. M. (1995). The alpha 2 beta 1 integrin: a collagen receptor on platelets and other cells. *Thromb Haemost*, , 74, 813-21.

[76] Savage, B, Almus-jacobs, F, & Ruggeri, Z. M. (1998). Specific synergy of multiple substrate-receptor interactions in platelet thrombus formation under flow. *Cell*, , 94, 657-66.

[77] Semple, J. W, & Freedman, J. (2010). Platelets and innate immunity. *Cell Mol Life Sci*, , 67, 499-511.

[78] Sheu, J. R, Hsiao, G, Lee, C, Chang, W, Lee, L. W, Su, C. H, & Lin, C. H. (2000a). Antiplatelet activity of Staphylococcus aureus lipoteichoic acid is mediated through a cyclic AMP pathway. *Thromb Res*, , 99, 249-58.

[79] Sheu, J. R, Lee, C. R, Lin, C. H, Hsiao, G, Ko, W. C, Chen, Y. C, & Yen, M. H. (2000b). Mechanisms involved in the antiplatelet activity of Staphylococcus aureus lipoteichoic acid in human platelets. *Thromb Haemost*, , 83, 777-84.

[80] Shiraki, R, Inoue, N, Kawasaki, S, Takei, A, Kadotani, M, Ohnishi, Y, Ejiri, J, Kobayashi, S, Hirata, K, Kawashima, S, & Yokoyama, M. (2004). Expression of Toll-like receptors on human platelets. *Thromb Res*, , 113, 379-85.

[81] Siboo, I. R, Chambers, H. F, & Sullam, P. M. (2005). Role of SraP, a Serine-Rich Surface Protein of Staphylococcus aureus, in binding to human platelets. *Infect Immun*, , 73, 2273-80.

[82] Siegel, I, & Cohen, S. (1964). Action of Staphylococcal Toxin on Human Platelets. *J Infect Dis*, , 114, 488-502.

[83] Tabuchi, A, & Kuebler, W. M. (2008). Endothelium-platelet interactions in inflammatory lung disease. *Vascul Pharmacol*, , 49, 141-50.

[84] Tang, Y. Q, Yeaman, M. R, & Selsted, M. E. (2002). Antimicrobial peptides from human platelets. *Infect Immun*, , 70, 6524-33.

[85] Thon, J. N, & Italiano, J. E. (2010). Platelet formation. *Semin Hematol*, , 47, 220-6.

[86] Thuny, F, Grisoli, D, Collart, F, Habib, G, & Raoult, D. (2012). Management of infective endocarditis: challenges and perspectives. *Lancet*, , 379, 965-75.

[87] Tzeng, D. Y, Deuel, T. F, Huang, J. S, & Baehner, R. L. (1985). Platelet-derived growth factor promotes human peripheral monocyte activation. *Blood*, , 66, 179-83.

[88] Varki, A. (1994). Selectin ligands. *Proc Natl Acad Sci U S A*, , 91, 7390-7.

[89] Wahl, S. M, Hunt, D. A, Wakefield, L. M, Mccartney-francis, N, Wahl, L. M, Roberts, A. B, & Sporn, M. B. (1987). Transforming growth factor type beta induces monocyte chemotaxis and growth factor production. *Proc Natl Acad Sci U S A*, , 84, 5788-92.

[90] Ward, J. R, Bingle, L, Judge, H. M, Brown, S. B, Storey, R. F, Whyte, M. K, Dower, S. K, Buttle, D. J, & Sabroe, I. (2005). Agonists of toll-like receptor (TLR)2 and TLR4 are unable to modulate platelet activation by adenosine diphosphate and platelet activating factor. *Thromb Haemost*, , 94, 831-8.

[91] Wilson, W, Taubert, K. A, Gewitz, M, Lockhart, P. B, Baddour, L. M, Levison, M, Bolger, A, Cabell, C. H, Takahashi, M, Baltimore, R. S, Newburger, J. W, Strom, B. L, Tani, L. Y, Gerber, M, Bonow, R. O, Pallasch, T, Shulman, S. T, Rowley, A. H, Burns, J. C, Ferrieri, P, Gardner, T, Goff, D, & Durack, D. T. (2007). Prevention of infective

endocarditis: guidelines from the American Heart Association: a guideline from the American Heart Association Rheumatic Fever, Endocarditis and Kawasaki Disease Committee, Council on Cardiovascular Disease in the Young, and the Council on Clinical Cardiology, Council on Cardiovascular Surgery and Anesthesia, and the Quality of Care and Outcomes Research Interdisciplinary Working Group. *J Am Dent Assoc*, 138, 739-45, 747-60.

[92] Yeaman, M. R, Tang, Y. Q, Shen, A. J, Bayer, A. S, & Selsted, M. E. (1997). Purification and in vitro activities of rabbit platelet microbicidal proteins. *Infect Immun*, , 65, 1023-31.

[93] Youssefian, T, Drouin, A, Masse, J. M, Guichard, J, & Cramer, E. M. (2002). Host defense role of platelets: engulfment of HIV and Staphylococcus aureus occurs in a specific subcellular compartment and is enhanced by platelet activation. *Blood*, , 99, 4021-9.

[94] Zhang, G, Han, J, Welch, E. J, Ye, R. D, Voyno-yasenetskaya, T. A, Malik, A. B, Du, X, & Li, Z. (2009). Lipopolysaccharide stimulates platelet secretion and potentiates platelet aggregation via TLR4/MyD88 and the cGMP-dependent protein kinase pathway. *J Immunol*, , 182, 7997-8004.

Chapter 4

History of Antimicrobial Prophylaxis Protocols for Infective Endocarditis Secondary to Dental Procedures

Inmaculada Tomás and
Maximiliano Álvarez-Fernández

Additional information is available at the end of the chapter

http://dx.doi.org/10.5772/56118

1. Introduction

For several decades, the haematogenous spread of bacteria from the oral cavity has been considered a decisive factor in the pathogenesis of 10% to 15% of episodes of infective endocarditis (IE), suggesting that certain dental procedures may represent a significant risk factor [1]. Nowadays, however, this statement has its detractors; their main argument is that not all patients with heart valves infected by bacteria that typically colonize ecological niches of the oral cavity have undergone dental procedures. Furthermore, there is little evidence to date on the genetic similarity between bacteria isolated from the heart valves, from the bloodstream, and from the oral cavity of patients with IE [2,3].

Apart from its possible involvement in the development of episodes of IE, bacteraemia of oral origin has become of particular interest in the past 2 decades because it has been associated with the progression of atherosclerosis and may thus be related to ischemic processes, although the mechanism of action has not yet been fully elucidated [4-6]. A number of published clinical studies have demonstrated an association between periodontal disease and cardiovascular disease [7-9], and oral bacteria have been detected on heart valves and in atherosclerotic plaques and aortic aneurysms [10-12].

In 1935, Okell and Elliot [13] were the first authors to detect bacteraemia caused by *Streptococcus* species (in 64% of cases) after performing dental extractions on 138 patients. A year later, Burket and Burn [14] inoculated pigmented *Serratia marcescens* into the gingival sulcus of 90 patients before performing dental extractions and they subsequently isolated this bacterium in 20% of post-manipulation blood cultures. Those results confirmed that microorganisms from the oral cavity could enter the bloodstream after dental extraction. Between the mid 1930s and the early 1950s, numerous studies were published on the prevalence of post-dental extraction bacteraemia, with figures that varied between 2% and 83% [15-19]. In the early 1930s there was a growing awareness of the need for IE prophylaxis in patients with valvular heart disease undergoing certain dental manipulations, and the first guidelines recommending the use of certain sulfonamides to prevent IE of oral origin were published at the end of that decade. This chapter first provides a review of development of antimicrobial prophylaxis protocols for IE secondary to dental procedures between 1930 and 1955. Since the American Heart Association (AHA) published its first guideline for the prevention of IE secondary to dental procedures in 1955, several international committees formed mainly of cardiologists, infectious diseases specialists and pharmacologists have drawn up different prophylactic regimens based on findings published in the scientific literature. In the second part of this chapter we therefore review the changes in IE prophylaxis in the guidelines published by the AHA and the British Society of Antimicrobial Chemotherapy (BSAC) between 1960 and 2009, as well as those recently drawn up by other societies. Those guidelines provide a description of the susceptible patient, the at-risk dental procedures, the influence of the anaesthetic technique applied in dental treatment, the antibiotic prophylaxis protocols (antibiotics of choice, dose and route of administration) and the use of antiseptic prophylaxis.

2. Development of antimicrobial prophylaxis protocols for infective endocarditis secondary to dental procedures: 1930 to 1955

In the early 1930s, Brown and Abrahamson [20,21] were 2 of the pioneers of the application of IE prophylaxis before performing certain dental manipulations in patients with valvular heart disease. Those investigators recommended the prophylactic use of autogenous vaccines. In 1938, Feldman and Trace [22] suggested cleaning and scraping the teeth before any manipulation in order to reduce contamination of the operative field; they performed only 1 or 2 dental extractions per session, and followed this by curettage and irrigation of the periodontal pockets with antiseptics. A year later, Elliott [23] proposed perialveolar cauterization of the gingiva as a prophylactic measure after dental extraction; this technique not only sterilized the sulcus but also sealed the gingival capillaries, preventing the entry of microorganisms into the bloodstream. The practice of dental extractions under local anaesthesia with epinephrine by the infiltration technique was also recommended, as some authors had shown that this type of anaesthetic applied in this way created a barrier, preventing vascular invasion by the bacterial inoculum [14,22]. Fish and Maclean [24] recommended that teeth be filled with cotton soaked in a paste of zinc oxide and oil of cloves and that this should be renewed every few days; those authors also recommended the administration of a dose of prontosil (azosulfamide) before a dental extraction, in addition to cauterization of the gingiva. However, Bender and Pressman [17] soon declared themselves contrary to the use of cauterization to prevent post-dental extraction bacteraemia, arguing that the teeth extracted in all the published series in which this technique was used were single rooted and a maximum of only 2 teeth were extracted in each session. According to those authors, cauterization of multirooted teeth damaged the adjacent periodontal tissues [17].

The first guideline for antibiotic prophylaxis for IE associated with dental manipulations in patients with valvular heart disease were soon developed and were based on the use of certain sulfonamides [25,26]. In 1939, Long and Bliss [27] published a book titled *The Clinical and Experimental Use of Sulfanilamide, Sulfapyridine and Allied Compounds*, in which they recommended the prophylactic administration of sulfanilamide to patients with rheumatic heart disease before performing dental extractions. In 1941, Kolmer and Tuft [28] drew up the most complete prophylactic guidelines published up to that time; those authors did not favour "massive dental extractions" and recommended not extracting more than 2 teeth in a single session; they also recommended the use of an autogenous streptococcal vaccine obtained from culture of the apical area of the first tooth extracted, which was to be administered before extraction of the following tooth. On the matter of antibiotic prophylaxis, those investigators proposed a regimen based on the use of 15 grains of sulfapyridine every 6 hours, starting 2 days before the manipulation and continuing for 2 or 3 days afterwards; they also endorsed the protocol for the prolonged administration of sulfonamides –previously proposed by Thomas et al [25]–for patients with acute rheumatic fever; that protocol consisted of the administration of 10 grains of sulfanilamide twice a day for a period that ran from November to June [28]. In 1941, Spink [29] indicated that sulfanilamide had to be administered between 8 and 12 hours before the dental manipulation in order to achieve a serum concentration of 7 mg/100 ml at the time of the manipulation. A year later, Budnitz et al [30] proposed a prophylactic protocol that consisted of an initial dose of 1 g of sulfapyridine followed by 0.5 g every 4 hours for 6 to 7 days, performing the dental extraction on the third or fourth day.

In 1943, Northrop and Crowley [31] were the first authors to evaluate the effect of the antibiotic sulfathiazole on the prevalence of post-dental extraction bacteraemia; their study group was formed of 73 patients who received 1 g of sulfathiazole every 4 hours, starting at 4 pm the day before the dental treatment and finishing at 12 noon the day of the procedure, 1 to 2 hours before the dental extraction. Blood samples were collected to perform the corresponding cultures at baseline and at 10 seconds and 10 minutes after the manipulation. All the baseline blood cultures and all those collected at 10 minutes after the dental extraction were negative, both in the controls and in individuals receiving antibiotic prophylaxis; however, at 10 seconds after the dental extraction, 13% of controls presented detectable bacteraemia compared to 4% of those who received antibiotic therapy (with blood levels of sulfathiazole of at least 3 mg/100 ml). These authors therefore concluded that a serum concentration of sulfathiazole of 4-5 mg/100 ml was effective for the prevention of post-dental extraction bacteraemia [31]. A year later, in the *Journal of Oral Surgery*, the same authors published another study based on the administration of a single dose of 5 g of sulfathiazole 3 hours before the dental manipulation, observing a reduction in the percentage of post-dental extraction bacteraemia from 16% to 4% [32]. Hopkins [16] and Budnitz et al [30], in their respective studies of patients at risk of IE, administered sulfanilamide or sulfapyridine before dental extraction; in both series all the post-dental extraction blood cultures were negative. In 1945, Bender and Pressman [17], in a study of the prevalence of post-dental extraction bacteraemia, created 3 randomly assigned study groups: a control group, a sulfanilamide group (this group was administered 4 doses of 1.35 g of the drug the previous day and 2 g 4 hours before the manipulation) and a cauterisation group (cauterisation of the free gingival border and of the full depth of the pocket was performed after the dental extraction). The mean serum levels of sulfanilamide were 7.5 mg/100 ml. In contrast to the results reported previously by other authors [16], the administration of sulfanilamide in this study did not reduce the prevalence of immediate post-dental extraction bacteraemia (83% in the control group *versus* 77% in the sulfanilamide group), although there was a detectable reduction in the number of positive blood cultures at 10 minutes after completion of the manipulation (33% in the control group *versus* 13% in the sulfanilamide group) and in the number of bacterial species isolated. Those authors indicated that the good results reported previously in the literature could be attributable to the absence of para-aminobenzoic acid (necessary to neutralise the sulfonamides) from the culture media used in some studies and based their findings mainly on the bacteriostatic action of this group of antibiotics [17].

In 1948, Hirsh et al [33] were the first authors to investigate the effect of penicillin on the prevalence of post-dental extraction bacteraemia. The study population was composed of a control group of 65 patients and a study group of 65 patients who received 600,000 IU of penicillin intramuscularly 3 to 4 hours before the dental extraction. Blood samples were collected immediately after the completion of surgery and at 10 and 30 minutes. Although the overall percentage of bacteraemia did not decline significantly (46% in controls *versus* 37% in the group that received penicillin), evaluation of only those cultures that were positive for streptococcal species showed a significant reduction in the prevalence of positive cultures in the group receiving prophylaxis compared to the control group (15% *versus* 34%), confirming that penicillin was effective in reducing the prevalence of streptococcal bacteraemia, although not bacteraemia caused by other microorganisms. Those authors speculated about 2 possible mechanisms of action of penicillin in the prevention of bacteraemia secondary to dental extractions: the first was that the penicillin present in the blood destroyed the microorganisms that reached the bloodstream, and the second that the antibiotic could inhibit bacterial growth in the oral cavity, thus reducing the size of the inoculum before vascular invasion occurred [33]. In another study on the efficacy of penicillin in the prevention of post-dental extraction bacteraemia published the same year, Glaser et al [34] administered 50,000 IU of penicillin intramuscularly every 2 hours for 24 hours prior to dental extraction, administering the final injection approximately 20 minutes before the manipulation. They then determined the sensitivity to penicillin of the microorganisms isolated from the blood cultures of patients who received the antibiotic therapy. In that study, prophylaxis with penicillin significantly reduced the prevalence of post-dental extraction bacteraemia (by 25%), as well as the number of bacteria isolated: there was a predominance of α-haemolytic streptococci in the control group (81% *versus* 29% in the group that received penicillin) and the majority of streptococci isolated in the penicillin group were non-haemolytic. However, none of the microorganisms isolated in the subjects who received prophylaxis were resistant to penicillin, confirming that this was not the cause of onset of the bacteraemia. Two very interesting findings of that study were that prophylaxis with penicillin was more effective in patients with periodontal disease and in those in whom only a single dental extraction was performed. Finally, those authors described a third mechanism of action of penicillin in the prevention of IE, the inhibition of bacterial growth after implantation of the microorganisms on the endocardium and before the resulting disease became clinically detectable [34]. Rhoads and Schram [35] evaluated the efficacy of penicillin and a new sulfonamide, 3,4-dimethyl-5-sulfanilamidoisoxazole (Gantrosan), for the prevention of post-dental extraction bacteraemia. Based on their optimal results, those authors were emphatic in their indication of the need to administer antibiotic therapy prior to performing dental extractions in patients with valvular heart disease [35].

The book on oral surgery published by Thoma in 1948 [36] was the first to include antibiotic prophylaxis prior to oral surgical procedures in patients with heart disease, although no specific regimen was described. In the first edition of Archer's classic book on oral surgery published in 1952 [37], a complex prophylactic regimen was described based on the administration of an injection of procaine penicillin G the day before oral surgery and an injection of crystalline penicillin G 30 minutes before the procedure, followed by an injection of procaine penicillin G once a day for 3 days and an injection of bicillin together with the final injection of procaine penicillin G. A very similar antibiotic prophylaxis regimen appeared in another book on oral surgery published by Mead in 1954 [38], but the penicillin was limited to 3 doses: one the day before, one 20 to 30 minutes before the manipulation and the final one the day after the intervention.

In 1955, the Committee on Prevention of Rheumatic Fever and IE of the AHA, which at that time was formed exclusively by 7 physicians, developed the first prophylactic protocol for use in patients with IE undergoing dental procedures [39]. This protocol was recommended in patients with congenital or rheumatic heart disease who were undergoing dental extractions or other manipulations that affected the gingival tissues. The AHA experts stated that the aim of prophylaxis was to make high concentrations of the antibiotic available at the time of the manipulation and to maintain the presence of the drug in the bloodstream for several days in order to eliminate any bacteria that had adhered to the heart valves during the bacteraemic episode. The method chosen was an intramuscular injection of a dose of 600,000 IU of aqueous penicillin and 600,000 IU of procaine penicillin dissolved in oil with 2% aluminium monostearate administered 30 minutes before the dental procedure. Alternatively (although less desirable), they proposed the oral administration of 250,000-500,000 IU of penicillin 30 minutes before each meal and before bedtime, starting 24 hours before the dental treatment and continuing for 5 days afterwards, and with an extra dose of 250,000 IU of penicillin immediately prior to the manipulation. For patients with a history of allergy to penicillin, the AHA recommended the use of other antibiotics such as oxytetracycline, chlortetracycline or erythromycin for 5 days, with administration starting the day before dental treatment [39].

3. Development of antimicrobial prophylaxis protocols for infective endocarditis secondary to dental procedures: 1960 to 2009

Since the AHA published its first protocol for the prevention of IE associated with dental procedures, numerous expert committees in different countries have drawn up different prophylactic regimens, many of which have subsequently been revised and modified based on subsequent epidemiological and clinical studies (prevalence of bacteraemia secondary to dental procedures, studies of the efficacy of antibiotic and antiseptic prophylaxis, pharmacokinetics of antibiotic prophylaxis, antimicrobial sensitivity of isolates identified in post-dental manipulation blood cultures) and on animal experimentation [40].

The AHA has published 9 IE prophylaxis protocols, the latest revision being in 2007 [39,41-48]. The BSAC published its first antibiotic prophylaxis regimen for IE in 1982; this was revised and modified in 1986, 1990, 1992 and 2006 [49-53]. The European Society of Cardiology (ESC), together with the group of experts of the International Society of Chemotherapy published a European Consensus on IE prophylaxis in 1995 [54]. In 2004, the ESC and the British Cardiac Society (BCS), in association with the Royal College of Physicians (RCP) of London, drew up guidelines for the prevention of IE associated with dental procedures [55,56]. In 2008, the National Institute for Clinical Excellence (NICE) of the United Kingdom published clinical guidelines entitled "Prophylaxis against IE: antimicrobial prophylaxis against IE in adults and children undergoing interventional procedures" [57]. In that document, the NICE reviewed 4 clinical guidelines on the prevention of IE, including those published by the BSAC in 2006 and the AHA in 2007. The NICE also reviewed the available evidence on the principal issues of IE of oral origin and reported their conclusions. In 2009, the Task Force of the ESC published a new guideline on the prevention, diagnosis and treatment of IE [58].

3.1. Susceptible patients

In its 2 protocols published in the 1960s on the prevention of IE associated with dental procedures, the AHA defined subjects considered to be at risk of IE as those with rheumatic heart disease or congenital heart disease [41,42]. In the early seventies, the AHA emphasised that IE represented one of the most serious cardiac complications as it was associated with a high morbidity and mortality, though it recognised that it was impossible to predict which patients with cardiac abnormalities were susceptible to developing IE after interventions (including those performed in the dental setting) [43]. However, they added patients with a past history of IE, including those with no detectable cardiac abnormalities, to the list of patients considered to be at risk of IE. For the first time, the AHA indicated that patients who were candidates for cardiac surgery should undergo an exhaustive dental examination in order to perform all necessary treatments in the weeks prior to the operation, with the aim of reducing the risk of postoperative IE. After cardiac surgery, patients would remain indefinitely in the category labelled at risk of IE (particularly those with prosthetic valves) and would therefore be candidates for antibiotic prophylaxis. In the opinion of the AHA, patients with atrial septal secundum defects repaired surgically by direct suturing, without the need for a prosthetic patch, and patients who had undergone surgical repair of a patent ductus arteriosus were not at risk of IE; in the AHA's opinion, those patients would only need to receive antibiotic prophylaxis for dental treatment performed during the first 6 months after cardiac surgery [43].

Five years later, in its new guideline, the AHA pointed out that, despite advances in antimicrobial chemotherapy and cardiovascular surgery, IE continued to be associated with a significant morbidity and mortality [44]. For the first time, this Association listed those cardiac alterations considered to carry a risk of IE and in which the administration of antibiotic prophylaxis was indicated; the list included congenital heart disease, acquired valve disease (rheumatic fever), idiopathic hypertrophic subaortic stenosis, mitral valve prolapse with insufficiency and prosthetic valves, but not the presence of a secundum atrial septal defect. The AHA stated that mitral valve prolapse was associated with a relatively low incidence of IE and that the use of prophylaxis in these patients was therefore controversial. Antibiotic prophylaxis was not recommended for patients after coronary artery surgery, the insertion of pacemakers, those on renal dialysis with arteriovenous fistulae or hydrocephalic patients with ventriculoatrial shunts, although the it was added that "*It will be the physician or dentist who takes the final decision about whether the patient requires the administration of antibiotic prophylaxis*" [44].

In the first BSAC guideline on the prevention of IE secondary to dental procedures, patients considered to be at risk of IE included those with alterations of the endocardium due to congenital or acquired disease, those with valvular heart disease and those with prosthetic heart valves [49]. In 1984, the AHA stated that certain patients, such as those with prosthetic heart valves or surgically constructed systemic-pulmonary shunts, presented a higher risk of IE than patients with other heart conditions. This was the first guideline to include a discussion of the action to be taken in patients who were anticoagulated with heparin or dicoumarin derivatives, stating that the antibiotic prophylaxis should be administered intravenously or orally, and that intramuscular injections should be avoided because of the risk of causing haematomas [45].

In 1990, the AHA listed the heart conditions that did and did not require antibiotic prophylaxis [46]. On the subject of heart transplant patients, the AHA briefly commented that some experts considered these patients to be at risk of IE. In the case of patients with severe renal dysfunction, it was suggested that the second dose of antibiotic (gentamycin or vancomycin) proposed in some regimens should be omitted or modified [46]. Concerning the controversy over valve prolapse, in 1990, the BSAC gave its first opinion in favour of prophylaxis in mitral valve prolapse if the prolapse was associated with a systolic murmur [51].

The intense debate about IE prophylaxis that developed during the European Symposium held in Lyon in 1994 led an international group of experts to draw up a consensus protocol jointly with the Working Group on Valvular Heart Disease of the ESC [54]. The guideline was published in 1995 and it listed the heart conditions that required prophylaxis, establishing for the first time the conditions or diseases that were considered to carry a high risk of IE, such as prosthetic heart valves, cyanotic congenital heart disease and previous episodes of IE. The controversy concerning the administration of antibiotic prophylaxis in cases of mitral stenosis without valve incompetence was also discussed [54].

In 1997, the AHA adopted a more conservative attitude, admitting that the incidence of IE secondary to medico-surgical interventions in patients with cardiac abnormalities was low [47]. It was suggested that the indication for antibiotic prophylaxis should be conditioned by a number of factors such as the degree of risk of IE associated with the patient's specific cardiac abnormality, the probability that the procedure performed might cause bacteraemia, possible adverse reactions to the recommended antibiotics and the cost-benefit relationship of the prophylactic regimens. One of the important novelties introduced by the AHA was the differentiation between cardiac diseases with distinct levels of risk of developing IE (as had previously been done by the ESC in the European Consensus of 1995), and consideration of the associated morbidity and mortality (Table 1) [47].

PROPHYLAXIS RECOMMENDED	PROPHYLAXIS NOT RECOMMENDED
HIGH RISK OF IE	**LOW RISK OF IE**
-Valve prostheses	-Isolated secundum atrial septal defect
-Previous episodes of IE	-Surgically repaired structural heart defects (after 6 months)[c]
-Cyanotic congenital heart disease[a]	-Previous coronary artery bypass graft surgery
-Surgically constructed systemic-pulmonary shunts or conduits	-Physiological, functional or innocent heart murmurs[d]
MODERATE RISK OF IE	-History of Kawasaki's disease without valve dysfunction
-Structural heart defects[b]	-History of rheumatic fever without valve dysfunction
-Acquired valve disease (e.g. due to rheumatic disease)	-Cardiac pacemakers or defibrillators
-Hypertrophic obstructive cardiomyopathy	
-Mitral valve prolapse with regurgitation and/or thickened leaflets	

a- Including isolated ventricular defects, transposition of the great vessels and tetralogy of Fallot; b- Including ventricular septal defect, bicuspid aortic valve, primum atrial septal defects, patent ductus arteriosus and coarctation of the aorta; c- Including atrial and ventricular septal defects and patent ductus arteriosus; d- If the precise nature of the murmur is not known, specialist opinion should be sought.

Table 1. Classification of patients at risk of IE: AHA guideline (1997) [47].

The AHA also defined the profile of the patient with mitral valve prolapse in whom prophylaxis should be given as male, over 45 years of age, with mitral valve thickening and/or regurgitation. If the patient required emergency dental treatment and it was not known whether or not regurgitation secondary to the prolapse was present, the AHA recommended antibiotic prophylaxis. The AHA also stated that, whilst auscultation enabled innocent cardiac murmurs to be defined clearly in paediatric patients, their diagnosis in adults required complementary studies, such as echocardiography. Finally, the AHA reiterated that many professionals classified heart transplant recipients as having a moderate risk of IE indefinitely, as they were patients with a particular tendency to develop valve dysfunction (particularly during episodes of rejection) and because they were usually on immunosuppressants; these patients should therefore receive antibiotic prophylaxis [47].

In the guideline proposed by the ESC in 2004 [55], the classification of at-risk patients was similar to that published previously by the AHA in 1997 [47]. For the ESC, the classification represented a class I recommendation (when there is evidence and/or general agreement that a certain treatment or diagnostic approach is beneficial, useful or effective) with level C evidence (when there is expert consensus based on clinical trials or investigations). For the first time, the ESC added a number of so-called non-cardiac conditions in which antibiotic prophylaxis should be given: conditions that favour the development of nonbacterial thrombotic vegetations, those which compromise immune function and/or local non-immune defence mechanisms in the host and advanced age [55].

In 2004, the BSC and RCP indicated that the risk of developing IE varied according to the underlying cardiac abnormality and that, in the case of congenital heart disease, it depended on the haemodynamic repercussions of the condition and whether surgical treatment was palliative or curative [56]. To reflect these differences in susceptibility to IE, the experts established 3 risk groups (Table 2). The principal differences to be found on comparison with the classifications of at-risk patients published previously by the AHA [47] and ESC [55] were that mitral valve prolapse with regurgitation and/or thickening of the leaflets was incorporated into the high-risk group and that prophylaxis was recommended up to 12 months after atrial septal defect/patent foramen ovale (ASD/PFO) catheter-based closure procedures and only for the first 6 months after heart and/or lung transplant [56]. The BSC and RCP also recommended that all patients at risk of IE should have a card with the following information: type of cardiac lesion, degree of risk of developing IE, history of penicillin allergy, the prophylactic regimen that should be administered, and name and telephone number of the cardiologist [56].

PROPHYLAXIS RECOMMENDED	PROPHYLAXIS NOT RECOMMENDED
HIGH RISK OF IE	**LOW RISK OF IE**
-Prosthetic heart valves	-Pulmonary stenosis
-Previous episodes of IE	-Surgically repaired structural heart defects[c]
-Cyanotic congenital heart disease	-Post Fontan or Mustard procedure with no residual murmur or defect
-Transposition of the great vessels	-Isolated *secundum* atrial septal defect[d]
-Tetralogy of Fallot	-Previous coronary artery bypass surgery
-Gerbode's defect	-Mitral valve prolapse without regurgitation
-Surgically constructed systemic-pulmonary shunts or conduits	-Innocent heart murmurs[e]
-Mitral valve prolapse with clinical repercussion[a]	-Cardiac pacemakers or defibrillators[f]
MODERATE RISK OF IE	-Coronary artery stent implantation
-Acquired valve disease (e.g. due to rheumatic heart disease)	-Heart and/or lung transplant[g]
-Aortic stenosis	
-Aortic regurgitation	
-Mitral regurgitation	
-Structural heart defects[b]	
-Hypertrophic obstructive cardiomyopathy	
-Subaortic membrane	

a- Presence of mitral valve regurgitation and/or thickening of the valves; b- Including ventricular septal defects, bicuspid aortic valve, primum atrial septal defects, patent ductus arteriosus, aortic root replacement, coarctation of the aorta, atrial septal aneurysm and patent foramen ovale; c- Including atrial septal defect, ventricular septal defect and patent ductus arteriosus; d- Antibiotic prophylaxis recommended up to 12 months after catheter closure of ASD/PFO; e- If the precise nature of the murmur is not known, the opinion of a cardiologist should be sought; in emergency situations, even if the possible repercussion of the murmur is not known, prophylaxis may be administered for certain dental procedures; f- With the exception of patients considered to have a moderate or high risk of IE, in whom antibiotic prophylaxis is recommended; g- Antibiotic prophylaxis is recommended for the first 6 months after surgery.

Table 2. Classification of patients at risk of IE: BCS and RCP (London) guideline (2004) [56].

In recent years, the updated guidelines published by the BSAC [53], the AHA [48], the NICE [57] and the ESC [58] have limited prophylaxis to high-risk patients, but the cardiac conditions included by each Expert Committee differ (Table 3). For example, according to the latest AHA guideline, IE prophylaxis for dental procedures should be recommended only for patients with underlying cardiac conditions associated with the highest risk of adverse outcome from IE. The conditions included in the list were prosthetic heart valves, previous IE, congenital heart disease (unrepaired defect, repaired defect with residual alterations and the first 6 months after complete repair of a defect) and heart transplant recipients who develop valve disease [48]. Although the AHA guideline recommended prophylaxis in heart transplant recipients who developed valve disease, the ESC stated that such a recommendation was not supported by strong evidence. In addition, although the risk of an adverse outcome was high when IE occurred in transplant patients, the probability of IE of oral origin was extremely low in these patients. Consequently, the ESC did not recommend prophylaxis in such situations [58]. The ESC recommended prophylaxis for cardiac conditions associated with the highest risk of IE (the list is similar to the one proposed by the AHA, except for heart transplant) based on a Class IIa recommendation (weight of evidence/opinion is in favour of usefulness/efficacy) and Level C evidence (consensus of opinion of the experts and/or small studies, retrospective studies, registries)[58]. The NICE also included other cardiac conditions at risk of IE, such as acquired valve disease with stenosis or regurgitation and hypertrophic cardiomyopathy [57].

In our opinion, this lack of consensus could provoke conflicting situations for clinicians at the time of identifying high-risk patients requiring antibiotic prophylaxis, and this could have medico-legal repercussions. However, if a clinician takes into account all the high-risk cardiac conditions defined each of the Expert Committees, there would be no omissions from the group of at-risk patients requiring antibiotic prophylaxis compared with previous IE prophylaxis protocols [59].

3.2. At-risk dental procedures

In 1960, the AHA stated that the dental procedures in which prophylaxis was indicated were dental extractions and gingival treatments, specifying that these procedures frequently caused transient bacteraemia and that the bacteraemia was more intense in patients with oral infections. They also admitted that certain normal activities such as toothbrushing and chewing gave rise to bacteraemia, although of lower intensity [41].

In 1972, a dentist, Dean Millard, was incorporated for the first time onto the AHA panel of experts; this led to recognition of the importance of a good oral health status in minimising the risk of developing IE of oral aetiology. The administration of antibiotic prophylaxis was recommended before performing any dental procedure associated with the potential for causing bacteraemia, the intensity of which depended on the magnitude of the procedure, the degree of the trauma to the gingival tissues and the presence of infection. Prophylaxis was therefore recommended for any dental procedure that caused gingival bleeding [43]. Five years later, the AHA recognised the impossibility of predicting which dental procedures could be responsible for causing IE. Antibiotic prophylaxis was recommended for treatments that can

PROPHYLAXIS RECOMMENDED	
BSAC, 2006	**AHA, 2007/ESC, 2009**
-Previous episodes of IE -Prosthetic heart valve -Surgically constructed systemic or pulmonary shunt or conduit	-Previous episodes of IE -Prosthetic heart valve -Congenital heart disease (CHD)[a] Unrepaired cyanotic CHD, including palliative shunts and conduits First 6 months after complete repair of a congenital heart defect with prosthetic material or device, whether placed by surgery or by catheter intervention[b] Repaired congenital heart defect with residual defects at the site or adjacent to the site of a prosthetic patch or prosthetic device (which inhibits endothelialisation) -Heart transplant recipients who develop valve disease[c]
NICE, 2008	
-Previous episodes of IE -Prosthetic heart valve -Acquired valve disease with stenosis or regurgitation -Structural congenital heart disease, including surgically corrected or palliated structural conditions, but excluding isolated atrial septal defect, fully repaired ventricular septal defect or fully repaired patent ductus arteriosus, and closure devices that are judged to be endothelialised -Hypertrophic cardiomyopathy	

a- Except for the conditions listed above, antibiotic prophylaxis is no longer recommended for any other form of CHD; b- Prophylaxis is recommended because endothelialisation of prosthetic material can take up to 6 months after the procedure; c- Although the AHA guideline recommend prophylaxis in heart transplant recipients who develop valve disease, the ESC Task Force does not recommend prophylaxis in such situations.

Table 3. High-risk cardiac conditions requiring antibiotic prophylaxis for IE: guidelines of the BSAC (2006), the AHA (2007), the NICE of the United Kingdom (2008) and the ESC (2009) [48,53,57,58].

cause gingival bleeding, such as scaling, but not for procedures such as the adjustment of orthodontic appliances and the exfoliation of primary teeth [44].

In the first guideline for the prevention of IE published by the BSAC in 1982, antibiotic prophylaxis was recommended exclusively for dental extractions, scaling and root planing and periodontal surgery [49]. In 1986, the AHA confirmed that certain dental procedures such as dental extractions were associated with a higher frequency of significant bacteraemia than other treatments [50]. In 1990, the AHA reported that bacteraemia secondary to dental procedures did not persist for more than 15 minutes after completion of the procedure. However, their Committee reiterated the importance of maintaining an optimal oral health status in patients considered to be at risk of IE. On this matter, dentists were encouraged to minimise gingival inflammation. Curiously, the AHA also discussed the need to control the fit of dental prostheses in edentulous patients as there was a possibility of developing bacteraemia because of mucosal ulceration due to poorly fitting prostheses [46]. For its part, the BSAC, in 1992, pronounced for the first time against the use of intraligamental local anaesthesia in patients considered to be at risk of IE [52].

In 1995, the ESC declared that dental treatment constituted the principle risk factor for IE and that all procedures should therefore be performed under antibiotic prophylaxis, with the exception of superficial fillings and supragingival prosthetic preparations. However, the ESC recognised that although at-risk dental procedures led to a high prevalence of bacteraemia, this was not predictive of the risk of developing IE. In this context, the duration of the procedure could represent a possible conditioning factor [54].

In its guideline published in 1997, the AHA listed the dental procedures that required antibiotic prophylaxis and those in which this was not necessary (Table 4) [47].

PROPHYLAXIS RECOMMENDED	PROPHYLAXIS NOT RECOMMENDED
-Dental extractions	-Restorative dentistry (operative and prosthodontic) with or without retraction cord
-Periodontal procedures[a]	-Non-intraligamental anaesthetic injections
-Placement of implants and reimplantation of avulsed teeth	-Intracanal post placement and build-up
-Endodontal instrumentation or periapical surgery	-Placement of a rubber dam
-Placement of subgingival antibiotic fibres or strips	-Removal of sutures
-Initial placement of orthodontic bands	-Placement of removable prosthetic or orthodontic appliances
-Intraligamental anaesthetic injections	-Intra-oral impressions
-Cleaning of teeth or implants[b]	-Fluoride treatments
	-Intra-oral radiographs
	-Orthodontic appliance adjustment
	-Exfoliation of primary teeth

a- Including surgery, root planing and scaling, probing and maintenance; b- When bleeding is anticipated.

Table 4. Dental procedures and antibiotic prophylaxis in patients with a high or moderate risk of IE: AHA guideline (1997) [47].

In general, as in previous protocols, antibiotic prophylaxis was recommended for dental procedures associated with gingival bleeding but it was not recommended for restorative dental procedures (with or without gingival retraction), the placement of a rubber dam or the removal of sutures. Although the possibility of developing bacteraemia secondary to traumatic ulcers caused by poorly fitting prostheses had previously been included, the AHA no longer recommended prophylaxis in edentulous patients during the fitting of complete prostheses [47].

In 2004, in agreement with previous guidelines [47,52,54], the ESC once again recommended antibiotic prophylaxis for *"dental treatments that caused gingival or mucosal trauma"* [55]. In contrast, the BCS and the RCP modified certain aspects concerning bacteraemia of oral origin [56]. First, they excluded the concept of "*procedures that cause bleeding*" as a criterion for the indication for antibiotic prophylaxis in patients at risk of IE; they also re-evaluated the definition of "*significant bacteraemia*" which, according to their new interpretation, was defined as "*bacteraemia secondary to a dental procedure that was statistically significant with respect to the bacteraemia present under basal conditions (prior to any manipulation)*". Considering these new provisions, the indication for prophylaxis included not only surgical procedures such as dental extractions or mucoperiosteal flaps but also other less traumatic procedures such as the placement of a rubber dam, matrices, wedges or retraction cords (Table 5) [56]. Although that Committee recognised the existence of bacteraemia secondary to activities considered to be physiological (such as toothbrushing), it also recognised the impossibility of administering prophylaxis for such practices due to the high risk of potentiating the development of bacterial resistance [56].

In 2006, the BSAC summarized the indications for antibiotic prophylaxis for high-risk patients stating that it should be given for "*all dental procedures involving dento-gingival manipulation or endodontics*" [53]. According to the latest AHA and ESC guidelines, prophylaxis was recommended for all dental procedures that involved manipulation of gingival tissues or the periapical region of teeth or perforation of the oral mucosa. This included procedures such as biopsies, suture removal and placement of orthodontics bands, but it did not include routine anaesthetic injections through non-infected tissue, taking dental radiographs, placement of removable prosthodontic or orthodontic appliances, placement of orthodontic brackets, or adjustment of orthodontic appliances [48,58]. The dental procedures with the highest risk of IE and for which prophylaxis was recommended were associated with a Class IIa recommendation (weight of evidence/opinion is in favour of usefulness/efficacy) and Level C evidence (consensus of opinion of the experts and/or small studies, retrospective studies, registries) [58]. There are other events for which prophylaxis was not recommended, such as shedding of deciduous teeth and trauma to the lips or oral mucosa [48].

In the latest guidelines published by the BSAC, the AHA, the NICE of the United Kingdom, and the ESC, the emphasis for the cause of IE shifted from procedure-related bacteraemia to cumulative bacteraemia due to everyday oral activities [48,53,57,58]. The NICE considered that it was biologically implausible that a dental procedure would lead to a greater risk of IE than regular toothbrushing. On the other hand, even some expert committee guidelines concurred with the premise "*Maintenance of optimal oral hygiene and periodontal health may reduce the incidence of bacteraemia of oral origin and, in the context of a dental procedure, is more important than prophylactic antibiotics to reduce the risk of IE*" [48,58].

The NICE has adopted a drastic stance in this respect, issuing the statement that "*antibiotic prophylaxis for IE is not recommended in individuals undergoing dental procedures*" [58]. Recently, following the introduction in March 2008 of a clinical guideline from NICE recommending the cessation of antibiotic prophylaxis in the United Kingdom, Thornhill et al [60] quantified the change in the prescription of antibiotic prophylaxis to patients at risk of IE undergoing invasive dental procedures and looked for any concurrent change in the incidence of IE. Despite a 78.6% reduction in the prescription of antibiotic prophylaxis after the introduction of the NICE guideline, that study detected no large increase in the incidence of cases of IE or of IE-related deaths over the following 2 years. Those authors concluded that ongoing data monitoring was

TYPE OF PROCEDURE	PROPHYLAXIS RECOMMENDED	PROPHYLAXIS NOT RECOMMENDED
ORAL SURGERY	-Extraction of a single tooth -Extraction of multiple teeth -Mucoperiosteal flap for access to a tooth or lesion -Dental implants (as for mucoperiosteal flap)	-Incision and drainage of an abscess -Biopsy -Insertion of implants (transmucosal approach) -Exfoliation of primary teeth -Suture removal -Removal of surgical packs
PERIODONTICS	-Periodontal surgery -Gingivectomy -Root curettagea -Root planing (similar to curettage) -Placement of antibiotics in the gingival sulcusb -Rubber cup polishing -Oral irrigation with water	-Air polishing
ENDODONTICS	-Root canal instrumentation beyond the apex -Reimplantation of avulsed teeth[c]	-Root canal instrumentation (within the root canal) -Pulpotomy of primary molars -Pulpotomy of permanent molars[d]
ORTHODONTICS	-Placement of interproximal separators -Exposure of unerupted teeth	-Band placement and cementation -Band removal -Adjustment of fixed appliances -Taking alginate impressions
CONSERVATIVE DENTISTRY	-Placement of a rubber dam -Matrix band and wood wedge placement -Placement of a retraction cord	-Slow and fast drilling (without a rubber dam)
PREVENTIVE DENTISTRY		-Fossa and fissure sealing -Fluoride application
ANAESTHETIC TECHNIQUES	-Local intraligamental	-Local infiltrative -Local nerve block -General with oral intubation -General with nasal intubation -General with laryngeal mask
EXPLORATION TECHNIQUES	-Periodontal probing	-Dental examination with mirror and probe
DIAGNOSTIC TECHNIQUES	-Sialography	-Intra-oral radiographs -Extra-oral radiographs

a- Both supra and subgingival, with manual instrumentation or ultrasound; b- Although there are no studies on this subject, this procedure is very similar to the placement of a retraction cord; c- Antibiotic prophylaxis may be administered up to 2 hours after dental reimplantation; d- Although there are no studies on this subject, this procedure is very similar to pulpotomy of primary molars.

Table 5. Dental procedures and antibiotic prophylaxis in patients with a high or moderate risk of IE: BCS and RCP (London) guideline (2004) [56].

needed to confirm this observation supporting the NICE guideline and that further clinical trials should be performed to determine if antibiotic prophylaxis still has a role in protecting some patients at particularly high risk [60].

3.3. Anaesthetic technique

In 1960, the AHA recommended the administration of antibiotic prophylaxis for any surgical intervention (including those in the orofacial area) performed under general anaesthesia in patients considered to be at risk of IE [41]. However, in subsequent protocols published by the AHA, no specific observations were made with regard to the type of anaesthesia used [42-48].

The BSAC, on the other hand, specified for the first time in 1982 that when dental treatment was performed under general anaesthesia, special prophylactic protocols should be applied, also considering that "*If patients due to undergo a general anaesthesia have prosthetic heart valves and/or are allergic to penicillin and/or have received prolonged treatment with penicillin and/or have had* previous episodes of IE, their dental problems should be treated in a hospital environment" [49]. The BSAC has maintained that opinion in its protocols on IE prevention published in 1986, 1990 and 1992 [50-52]. In 1995, the ESC also included the anaesthetic technique among the factors to be taken into account when choosing the prophylactic regimen [54]. In the guideline published by the BCS and RCP in 2004, specific prophylaxis regimens were included for dental procedures performed under general anaesthesia [56].

In agreement with the AHA, the latest protocols of the BSAC and ESC on IE prevention recommend antibiotic prophylaxis irrespective of whether the dental procedure is performed under general or local anaesthesia [53,58].

3.4. Antibiotics of choice, dose and route of administration

In 1960, the AHA pronounced in favour of administering antibiotic prophylaxis from between 24 and 48 hours before the dental procedure, even in the absence of intraoral infections, in order to reduce the intensity of the post-manipulation bacteraemia [41]. However, in view of the problem of bacterial resistance, it was also suggested that prophylaxis could be administered immediately before the procedure. According to the AHA, the choice of one or other regimen depended on the professional, who should evaluate the probability of infection in order to decide when the prescription of antibiotics was indicated. In contrast to the guideline published in 1955 [39], the exclusively oral protocols were excluded in favour of intramuscular administration, although penicillin continued to be the antibiotic of choice; the prophylactic regimen consisted of several injections of penicillin from 2 days before up to 2 days after the session of dental treatment. A combined intramuscular-oral prophylactic regimen was also elaborated. For patients with a history of penicillin allergy, the AHA was the first to recommended erythromycin at doses of 250 mg orally 4 times a day (for adults and older children); in small children, the dose of erythromycin was of 20 mg/kg body-weight per day, divided into 3 or 4 doses, not exceeding a total dose of 1 g per day [41].

In 1965, the AHA stated that antibiotic prophylaxis should only be administered immediately before the dental procedure and on the subsequent days; this recommendation was based on the argument that penicillin did not sterilise the apical foci, and that its excessive use led to the selection of a resistant oral flora. The AHA also reduced the parenteral regimen to a single injection of several penicillins. In those cases in which the complete collaboration of the patient could be anticipated, an exclusively oral regimen of several doses of penicillin was proposed. Erythromycin was recommended for patients allergic to penicillin [42].

In 1972, the AHA modified its recommendations to include an increase in the initial doses of penicillin and erythromycin administered orally and the use of erythromycin in patients on prolonged treatments with penicillin, as penicillin-resistant *Streptococcus viridans* could predominate in their oral flora [43]. Five years later, the AHA suggested increasing the initial dose of the antibiotic even further in order to reach higher serum concentrations at the moment at which the microorganism entered the bloodstream [44]. However, they favoured the parenteral regimen, particularly in patients considered to be at high risk of IE. Two regimens were recommended: regimen A, based on the use of penicillin (erythromycin was recommended in patients allergic to penicillin) for parenteral-oral or exclusively oral administration, and regimen B, which combined penicillin and streptomycin (vancomycin and erythromycin for patients allergic to penicillin) for parenteral-oral administration. This latter protocol was reserved for patients with prosthetic heart valves, although patients with a good oral health status could receive the oral prophylaxis regimen for certain non-surgical dental procedures [44].

The BSAC, in its first guideline, suggested a single prophylactic regimen of a single dose of amoxicillin before the dental procedure for all patients considered to be at risk of IE (including patients with prosthetic heart valves) [49]. The BSAC substituted penicillin V, previously recommended by the AHA [44], with amoxicillin due to its more favourable pharmacokinetic and pharmacodynamic characteristics. Erythromycin stearate was the antibiotic of choice in patients allergic to penicillin but because this macrolide has lower activity than amoxicillin against some oral streptococci and showed a lower absorption after a single oral dose, they proposed a second dose 6 hours after completing the dental procedure. One quarter of the adult dose was recommended in children under 5 years of age and a half dose in those of 5 to 10 years of age [49]. In contrast to the AHA [44], the BSAC proposed a combined intramuscular-oral regimen in patients undergoing dental treatment under general anaesthesia. Special prophylactic regimens were proposed for patients being treated in the hospital environment; these regimens were based on the association of amoxicillin and gentamycin or, in patients unable to receive penicillin, a combination of vancomycin and gentamycin; the following doses were used in children under 10 years of age: amoxicillin, half the adult dose; gentamycin, 2 mg/kg body-weight; and vancomycin, 20 mg/kg body-weight [49].

In its protocol published in 1984, the AHA reduced the dose of the antibiotic after completion of the dental treatment, recommending the administration of penicillin V before the dental procedure and a second dose 6 hours after the first. In those patients in whom the oral route was not available, intramuscular penicillin G was proposed before the procedure and 6 hours later [45]. The AHA also showed a clear preference for the parenteral route in patients at high risk of IE and drew up a special regimen for these patients consisting of intramuscular or intravenous ampicillin and gentamycin, together with a second dose of penicillin V orally;

http://dx.doi.org/10.5772/56118

intravenous vancomycin was recommended for patients allergic to penicillin, eliminating the second dose of erythromycin [45].

In 1986, the BSAC suggested that vancomycin should be given by slow intravenous infusion over 60 minutes (instead of the previously recommended 30 minutes) to minimise adverse reactions such as episodes of hypotension caused by histamine release (red-man syndrome) [50]. As an alternative to the parenteral regimen proposed earlier, the BSAC proposed 2 oral regimens for patients without prosthetic heart valves undergoing dental treatment under general anaesthesia. The first was based on the administration of amoxicillin before anaesthetic induction followed by a second dose in the immediate postoperative period; the second regimen consisted of the combination of amoxicillin and probenecid administered before anaesthesia [50]. For the first time, the BSAC differentiated between patients with prosthetic heart valves and other patients considered to be at risk of IE, as the AHA [45] had done in its 1984 guideline, proposing specific oral prophylactic regimens for such patients undergoing dental treatment under local anaesthesia [50].

Differing from the BSAC guideline [50], the 1990 AHA guideline continued to favour regimens based on 2 doses. Of particular note amongst the novelties introduced in this protocol was the incorporation of amoxicillin as the antibiotic of choice for all groups at risk of IE [46], an approach that had been adopted by the BSAC in 1982 [49]. According to the AHA, amoxicillin, ampicillin and penicillin showed similar efficacy against α-haemolytic streptococci *in vitro* but amoxicillin reached higher serum concentrations due to its better gastrointestinal absorption. However, they also defended the use of penicillin V as a suitable alternative for prophylaxis in dental procedures. Erythromycin, in its ethylsuccinate or stearate salt preparations, continued to be the antibiotic of choice in patients allergic to penicillin, being administered 2 hours before the procedure to ensure high serum concentrations. For the first time, the AHA recommended the administration of clindamycin in patients intolerant to penicillin and erythromycin [46]. For patients unable to take oral medication, the AHA drew up a number of regimens for parenteral administration as alternatives to the standard protocol, proposing ampicillin (in patients not allergic to penicillin) and clindamycin (in penicillin-allergic patients) as the antibiotics of choice [46]. In contrast to the previous protocols [45], the AHA recommended the administration of the standard regimen to patients with prosthetic heart valves and other patients considered to be at high risk of IE (patients with a past history of IE and those with surgically constructed systemic-pulmonary shunts). However, recognising that some professionals preferred parenteral prophylaxis, they also drew up a special parenteral regimen for this type of patient [46].

The prophylactic protocol recommended by the BSAC in 1990 included a new option [51]. Due to the high prevalence of undesirable gastrointestinal effects caused by erythromycin, and based on the guideline published in 1984 by the Swiss Expert Committee for the prevention of IE [61], the BSAC proposed the administration of a single oral dose of 600 mg of clindamycin 1 hour before the procedure as an alternative in patients with penicillin allergy; the dose of clindamycin in children under 10 years of age was of 6 mg/kg body-weight [51]. In 1992, the BSAC definitively replaced erythromycin with clindamycin in patients allergic to penicillin, modifying the initial dose in children to 300 mg in those between 5 and 10 years of age and to 150 mg in those under 5 years [52]. Due to the high prevalence of adverse effects associated with vancomycin and its prolonged duration of administration (around 100 minutes), the BSAC drew up 2 alternative regimens for penicillin-allergic patients with a high risk of IE who were being treated in the hospital environment. One was based on the intravenous combination of teicoplanin and gentamycin (in children under 14 years of age the doses were teicoplanin, 6 mg /kg body-weight, and gentamycin, 2 mg/kg body-weight); and the other consisted of an intravenous infusion of clindamycin with a second dose 6 hours after the first. Finally, in patients undergoing dental treatment under general anaesthesia, the BSAC specified that prophylaxis with amoxicillin should be administered intravenously instead of intramuscularly, particularly in children [52].

In 1995, the ESC performed a critical review of the prophylaxis protocols drawn up by the different national committees, noting clear differences between countries, although all included a simple or standard regimen and another more complex regimen for use in special circumstances [54]. In general, the standard guidelines consisted of the oral administration of a single dose of antibiotic which, in the majority of countries, was amoxicillin. Some societies recommended the administration of a second dose, particularly in patients considered to be at high risk of IE. In patients allergic to the beta-lactams, the antibiotic of choice was clindamycin at doses between 300 mg and 600 mg, although some countries, for example, Holland and France, recommended other antibiotics such as erythromycin or pristinamycin [54]. The more complex regimens were based on the synergistic and prolonged effect provided by several doses of different antibiotics with the aim of increasing the safety margin in special situations. In an analysis performed by the ESC, it was found that the majority of protocols recommended ampicillin or amoxicillin by intravenous infusion followed by a second oral dose 6 hours later; there were only minor differences with respect to the doses used. Although some countries did not use the aminoglycosides, these were recommended in other countries in patients considered to be at high risk of IE. The most frequently used antibiotic of choice in patients allergic to penicillin was vancomycin by intravenous infusion; for some scientific societies, teicoplanin and clindamycin were possible antimicrobial alternatives [54]. According to the ESC, the choice of the most suitable prophylactic regimen should be based on the following considerations: the heart condition defined as carrying a risk of IE; the type, magnitude and duration of the dental procedure; and the type of anaesthesia used (local or general). The ESC therefore considered the possibility of individualising the antibiotic prophylaxis regimen in certain situations [54]. The oral regimen proposed by the ESC consisted of the administration of amoxicillin or clindamycin (in penicillin-allergic patients), whilst the combination of amoxicillin or ampicillin with gentamycin and a second dose of amoxicillin orally 6 hours later was recommended in the parenteral regimen. In patients allergic to penicillin, the association of vancomycin and gentamycin was recommended, administering a second dose of vancomycin by intravenous infusion 12 hours after the first dose [54].

The prophylactic protocol recommended by the AHA in 1997 is shown in Table 6 [47]. It is based on a single dose of amoxicillin administered orally 1 hour before the procedure. In this protocol, the dose of amoxicillin was reduced from 3 g to 2 g after confirming that this latter dose provided adequate serum levels of the drug over several hours and caused fewer adverse gastrointestinal effects. Accepting an approach that had been adopted by other societies several years earlier [49-52], the AHA recognised that the administration of a second dose of antibiotic was unnecessary, since the serum levels of the drug exceeded the minimum inhibitory concentra-

http://dx.doi.org/10.5772/56118

tions of many oral *Streptococcus* spp. and the antimicrobial activity of amoxicillin was prolonged (6 to 14 hours). In patients allergic to penicillin, the antibiotics of choice were clindamycin, cephalosporins (cefalexin or cefadroxil) or macrolides (azithromycin or clarithromycin), although the AHA specified that the cephalosporins should be avoided in patients with type 1 hypersensitivity to penicillin [47]. In patients unable to take oral medication or with problems of gastrointestinal absorption (independently of the IE risk category), the AHA drew up a regimen based on the use of intramuscular or intravenous ampicillin 30 minutes before the procedure. In penicillin-allergic patients in whom parenteral administration of the antibiotic was required, the recommended antibiotic was clindamycin phosphate and, in those patients not presenting type 1 hypersensitivity, was cefazolin. Although erythromycin was abandoned because of its gastrointestinal complications and its particular pharmacokinetic characteristics, the AHA indicated that "*Dentists who are used to prescribing this antibiotic successfully for prophylaxis may continue to use it*" [47].

STANDARD REGIMEN (ORAL)	
NOT ALLERGIC TO PENICILLIN	
ADULTS	CHILDREN
2 g of amoxicillin 1 h before tmt	50 mg/kg body-weight of amoxicillin 1 h before tmt
ALLERGIC TO PENICILLIN	
ADULTS	CHILDREN
A) 600 mg of clindamycin 1 h before tmt B) 2 g of cefalexin or cefadroxil 1 h before tmt[a] C) 500 mg of azithromycin or clarithromycin 1 h before tmt	A) 20 mg/kg body-weight of clindamycin 1 h before tmt B) 50 mg/kg body-weight of cefalexin or cefadroxil 1 h before tmt[a] C) 15 mg/kg body-weight of azithromycin or clarithromycin 1 h before tmt
PARENTERAL REGIMEN[b]	
NOT ALLERGIC TO PENICILLIN	
ADULTS	CHILDREN
2 g of ampicillin (IM or IV) 30 min before tmt	50 mg/kg body-weight of ampicillin (IM or IV) 30 min before tmt
ALLERGIC TO PENICILLIN	
ADULTS	CHILDREN
A) 600 mg of clindamycin (IV) 30 min before tmt B) 1 g of cefazolin (IM or IV) 30 min before tmt	A) 20 mg/kg body-weight of clindamycin (IV) 30 min before tmt B) 25 mg/kg body-weight of cefazolin (IM or IV) 30 min before tmt

tmt= treatment; min= minutes; h= hours; IM= intramuscular; IV=intravenous; mg= milligrams; g= grams; kg= kilograms.

a- The cephalosporins must not be administered to subjects with immediate hypersensitivity reactions to penicillin (urticaria, angioedema or anaphylaxis); b- This protocol is to be applied in patients unable to take the medication orally; the total dose in children should not exceed the adult dose.

Table 6. IE prophylaxis protocol for dental procedures: recommendation of the AHA (1997) [47].

In 2004, the ESC published a guideline on IE prophylaxis which were very similar to the 1997 guideline of the AHA [47], except that the use of cephalosporins in patients allergic to penicillin was excluded [55].

In the prophylaxis protocol for IE secondary to dental procedures drawn up by the BSC and RCP (London) in 2004, prophylaxis was reserved for patients with heart diseases included in the categories of high and moderate risk of IE, and the prophylactic regimens varied according to the type of anaesthesia used [56]. Oral prophylaxis regimens were to be administered in procedures performed under local anaesthesia and parenteral regimens for those performed under general anaesthesia (Tables 7 and 8) [56]. In contrast to the 1997 guideline of the AHA [47], the BCS and RCP also provided a special prophylactic regimen for patients with prosthetic heart valves and/or previous episodes of IE (Table 9) [56].

The most recent IE prophylaxis protocols published by the BSAC [53], the AHA [48] and the ESC [58] are very similar and are summarized in Tables 10 and 11. The most recent prophylactic protocol published by the AHA continues to recommend amoxicillin as the antibiotic of choice for oral prophylaxis. For individuals who are allergic to penicillins, the use of cephalexin or another first-generation oral cephalosporin, clindamycin, azithromycin or clarithromycin is recommended [48]. Because of possible cross-reactions, a cephalosporin must not be administered to patients with a history of anaphylaxis, angioedema or urticaria after treatment with any form of penicillin, including ampicillin or amoxicillin. Patients who are unable to tolerate an oral antibiotic may be treated with intramuscular or intravenous ampicillin, ceftriaxone or cefazolin. For penicillin-allergic patients who are unable to tolerate an oral agent, prophylaxis is recommended with parenteral cefazolin, ceftriaxone or clindamycin [48]. According to the ESC, the main aim of antibiotic prophylaxis in patients at risk of IE is to target the oral streptococci. The impact of increasing resistance of these pathogens on the efficacy of antibiotic prophylaxis is unclear. Fluoroquinolones and glycopeptides are not recommended because their efficacy has not been established and because of the potential induction of resistance [58].

It has been estimated that the number of cases of IE that result from dental interventions is very small. The AHA has therefore concluded that only an extremely small number of cases of IE will be prevented by antibiotic prophylaxis for dental procedures even if such prophylactic regimens are 100% effective [48]. According to the ESC, this observation leads to 2 conclusions: (i) IE prophylaxis can at best only protect a small proportion of patients; and (ii) the bacteraemia that causes IE in the majority of patients appears to derive from another source [58]. Finally, the AHA stated the need for prospective placebo-controlled studies of antibiotic prophylaxis for IE to evaluate its efficacy in IE prevention [48].

Reviewing the effect of antibiotic prophylaxis on the intensity and duration of bacteraemia following dental procedures, the NICE recently concluded that "*Antibiotic prophylaxis does not eliminate bacteraemia following dental procedures but some studies show that it does reduce the frequency of detection of post-procedure bacteraemia*" [57]. This conclusion was reached after analysis of a number of studies on the efficacy of antibiotic prophylaxis for the prevention of post-dental manipulation bacteraemia; those studies presented methodological differences with respect to the type of antibiotic used and the time and route of administration. These important differences make a comparison of the results between the different series inappropriate [59].

STANDARD REGIMEN (ORAL)	
NOT ALLERGIC TO PENICILLIN	
ADULTS 3 g of amoxicillin 1 h before tmt	CHILDREN OVER 10 YEARS OF AGE Adult dose CHILDREN BETWEEN 5 AND 10 YEARS OF AGE 1.5 g of amoxicillin 1 h before tmt CHILDREN UNDER 5 YEARS OF AGE 750 mg of amoxicillin 1 h before tmt
ALLERGIC TO PENICILLIN[a]	
ADULTS 600 mg of clindamycin 1 h before tmt	CHILDREN OVER 10 YEARS OF AGE Adult dose CHILDREN BETWEEN 5 AND 10 YEARS OF AGE 300 mg of clindamycin 1 h before tmt CHILDREN UNDER 5 YEARS OF AGE 150 mg of clindamycin 1 h before tmt
UNABLE TO TAKE ORAL MEDICATION[b]	
ADULTS 500 mg of azithromycin 1 h before tmt	CHILDREN OVER 10 YEARS OF AGE Adult dose CHILDREN BETWEEN 5 AND 10 YEARS OF AGE 300 mg of azithromycin 1 h before tmt CHILDREN UNDER 5 YEARS OF AGE 200 mg of azithromycin 1 h before tmt

h= hours; tmt= treatment; mg= milligrams; g= grams.

a- This protocol should also be used in patients who have received penicillin or another beta-lactam on more than 1 occasion in the previous month; b- In Great Britain, clindamycin is not available in oral suspension.

Table 7. IE prophylaxis protocol for dental procedures performed under local anaesthesia: recommendation of the BCS and RCP (London) (2004) [56].

PARENTERAL REGIMEN	
NOT ALLERGIC TO PENICILLIN	
ADULTS	CHILDREN OVER 10 YEARS OF AGE
2 g of amoxicillin or ampicillin (IV) during anaesthetic induction	Adult dose
	CHILDREN BETWEEN 5 AND 10 YEARS OF AGE
	500 mg of amoxicillin or ampicillin (IV) during anaesthetic induction
	CHILDREN UNDER 5 YEARS OF AGE
	250 mg of amoxicillin or ampicillin (IV) during anaesthetic induction
ALLERGIC TO PENICILLIN[a]	
ADULTS	CHILDREN OVER 10 YEARS OF AGE
300 mg of clindamycin (IV over 10 min) during anaesthetic induction	Adult dose
	CHILDREN BETWEEN 5 AND 10 YEARS OF AGE
150 mg of clindamycin (oral or IV) 6 h after the first dose	150 mg of clindamycin (IV over 10 min) during anaesthetic induction
	CHILDREN UNDER 5 YEARS OF AGE
	75 mg of clindamycin (IV over 10 min) during anaesthetic induction

min= minutes; h= hours; IV= intravenous; mg= milligrams; g= grams; kg= kilograms.

a-This protocol should also be used in patients who have received penicillin or another beta-lactam on more than 1 occasion in the previous month.

Table 8. IE prophylaxis protocol for dental procedures under general anaesthesia: recommendation of the BCS and RCP (London) (2004) [56].

PARENTERAL REGIMEN	
NOT ALLERGIC TO PENICILLIN	
ADULTS	CHILDREN OVER 10 YEARS OF AGE
2 g of amoxicillin + 1.5 mg/kg body-weight of gentamycin (IV) 30 min before tmt	Adult dose
	CHILDREN UNDER 10 YEARS OF AGE
1 g of amoxicillin (oral or IV) 6 h after the first dose	1 g of amoxicillin + 1.5 mg/kg body-weight of gentamycin (IV) 30 min before tmt
	Amoxicillin (oral) 6 h after the first dose
ALLERGIC TO PENICILLIN[a]	
ADULTS	CHILDREN OVER 10 YEARS OF AGE
1 g of vancomycin (IV over 2 h) + 1.5 mg/kg body-weight of gentamycin (IV) before tmt	Adult dose
	CHILDREN UNDER 10 YEARS OF AGE
	20 mg/kg body-weight of vancomycin (IV over 2 h) + 1.5 mg/kg body-weight of gentamycin (IV) before tmt

min= minutes; h= hours; tmt= treatment; IV= intravenous; mg= milligrams; g= grams; kg= kilograms.

a- This protocol should also be used in patients who have received penicillin or another beta-lactam on more than 1 occasion in the previous month.

Table 9. Parenteral IE prophylaxis protocol for patients with prosthetic heart valves and/or previous episodes of IE undergoing dental procedures under local or general anaesthesia: recommendations of the BCS and RCP (London) (2004) [56].

More than half of the studies published on antibiotic prophylaxis and post-dental extraction bacteraemia have investigated the efficacy of the penicillins. The results obtained in the majority of those studies confirmed the efficacy of these antibiotics in prevention, as bacteraemia did not develop in a significant number of patients (compared with the results obtained in patients not receiving antibiotic prophylaxis) [62,63]. However, there are fewer studies on the effect of the prophylactic administration of other antibiotics (clindamycin, azithromycin and cephalosporins) recommended for the prevention of post-dental extraction bacteraemia, and their results have not established whether these antibiotics are effective [62].

	STANDARD REGIMEN (ORAL)	
BSAC, 2006	**NOT ALLERGIC TO PENICILLIN**: 3 g of amoxicillin 1 h before tmt	
	ALLERGIC TO PENICILLIN: 600 mg of clindamycin 1 h before tmt	
	UNABLE TO TAKE ORAL MEDICATION[a] : 500 mg of azithromycin 1 h before tmt	
AHA, 2007	**NOT ALLERGIC TO PENICILLIN**:	2 g of amoxicillin 1 h before tmt
	ALLERGIC TO PENICILLIN:	2 g of cephalexin 1 h before tmt[b]
		600 mg of clindamycin 1 h before tmt
		500 mg of azithromycin or clarithromycin 1 h before tmt
ESC, 2009	**NOT ALLERGIC TO PENICILLIN**: 2 g of amoxicillin 30 min-1 h before tmt	
	ALLERGIC TO PENICILLIN: 600 mg of clindamycin 30 min-1 h before tmt	

tmt= treatment; min= minutes; h= hours; mg= milligrams; g= grams.

a- In Great Britain, clindamycin is not available in oral suspension; b- Cephalosporins must not be administered to subjects with immediate hypersensitivity reactions to penicillin (urticaria, angioedema or anaphylaxis).

Table 10. IE prophylaxis protocols (oral regimens) for dental procedures: recommendations of the BSAC (2006), the AHA (2007) and the ESC (2009) [48,53,58].

For children, the BSAC recommended amoxicillin (≥10 years, adult dose; ≥5-<10 years, 1.5 g; <5 years, 750 mg), clindamycin (≥10 years, adult dose; ≥5-<10 years, 300 mg; <5 years, 150 mg) or azithromycin (≥10 years, adult dose; ≥5-<10 years, 300 mg; <5 years, 200 mg). For children, the AHA recommended amoxicillin (50 mg/kg body-weight), clindamycin (20 mg/kg body-weight), cefalexin (50 mg/kg body-weight), or azithromycin or clarithromycin (15 mg/kg body-weight). For children, the ESC recommended amoxicillin (50 mg/kg body-weight) or clindamycin (20 mg/kg body-weight).

For children, the AHA and ESC recommended ampicillin or amoxicillin (50 mg/kg body-weight), clindamycin (20 mg/kg body-weight), or cephalexin, cefazolin or ceftriaxone (50 mg/kg body-weight).

For children, the BSAC recommended amoxicillin (≥10 years, 1 g; ≥5-<10 years, 500 mg; <5 years, 250 mg) or clindamycin (≥10 years, 300 mg; ≥5-<10 years, 150 mg; <5 years, 75 mg).

A second conclusion reached by the NICE was that "*It is not possible to determine the effect of antibiotic prophylaxis on the duration of bacteraemia*". Probably influenced by the idea that

	PARENTERAL REGIMEN	
BSAC, 2006	**NOT ALLERGIC TO PENICILLIN**: 1 g of amoxicillin (IV) just before tmt or at induction of anaesthesia **ALLERGIC TO PENICILLIN**: 300 mg of clindamycin (IV)[a] just before tmt or at induction of anaesthesia	
AHA, 2007	**NOT ALLERGIC TO PENICILLIN**:	2 g of ampicillin (IM or IV) 30 min before tmt
	ALLERGIC TO PENICILLIN:	1 g of cefazolin or ceftriaxone (IM or IV) 30 min before tmt[c] 600 mg of clindamycin (IM or IV) 30 min before tmt
ESC, 2009	**NOT ALLERGIC TO PENICILLIN**:	2 g of ampicillin (IV) 30 min-1 h before tmt
	ALLERGIC TO PENICILLIN:	2 g of cephalexin (IV) 30 min-1 h before tmt 1 g of cefazolin or ceftriaxone (IM or IV) 30 min before tmt[c] 600 mg of clindamycin (IV) 30 min-1 h before tmt

tmt= treatment; min= minutes; h= hours; IM= intramuscular; IV= intravenous; mg= milligrams; g= grams.

a- Given over at least 10 min; b- Given over 2 hours; c- Cephalosporins must not be administered to subjects with immediate hypersensitivity reactions to penicillin (urticaria, angioedema or anaphylaxis).

Table 11. IE prophylaxis protocols (parenteral regimens) for dental procedures: recommendations of the BSAC (2006), the AHA (2007) and the ESC (2009) [48,53,58].

bacteraemia secondary to dental procedures is of a transitory nature, few studies have been published on the effect of antibiotic prophylaxis on the duration of post-dental extraction bacteraemia [40]. On this question, the results of our research group have shown that the prophylactic administration of oral amoxicillin (2 g) significantly reduces the prevalence of bacteraemia at 15 minutes and 1 hour after completing dental extractions under general anaesthesia [62]. The conclusions reached by the NICE on the lack of efficacy of antibiotic prophylaxis for the prevention of bacteraemia following dental procedures are based on a small volume of published scientific evidence [59]. Further research should therefore be performed on the recommended antibiotics regimens for IE prophylaxis, analysing the influence of the choice of antibiotic and the time and route of administration, and also on new antibiotic protocols [40].

Antibiotic administration does carry a small risk of anaphylaxis [58]. However, no case of fatal anaphylaxis has been reported in the literature after the oral administration of amoxicillin for IE prophylaxis [63]. Widespread and often inappropriate use of antibiotics may result in the emergence of resistant microorganisms [58], but the extent to which antibiotic use for IE prophylaxis could be implicated in the general problem of resistance is unknown [64].

3.5. Antiseptics

In 1977, the AHA suggested for the first time performing disinfection of the gingival sulcus as a complement to antibiotic prophylaxis, although they recommended caution in the use of oral irrigators in patients considered to be at risk of IE, particularly in the presence of deficient oral hygiene habits [44]. This approach was also adopted by the BSAC en 1982 [49], when it recommended the application of antiseptics at the gingival margins in addition to the prophylactic administration of antibiotics prior to dental manipulations.

In 1990, the AHA recommended the application of chlorhexidine or other antiseptics (povidone iodine or a combination of iodine and glycerine) for 3 to 5 minutes around the tooth—a proposal also supported by the BSAC at that time [51]—before performing dental extractions in patients considered to be at high risk of IE and/or with deficient oral hygiene [46]. Two years later, the BSAC specified the form of presentation and the concentration of chlorhexidine to be used before starting a dental procedure: 1% gel at the gingival margin or 0.2% mouthwash for 5 minutes [52].

In the European Consensus of 1995, the application of antiseptics was once again recommended as a complementary measure in addition to antibiotic prophylaxis [54]. In its 1997 recommendations, the AHA recognised the need to use antiseptic mouthwashes (chlorhexidine or povidone iodine) prior to a dental manipulation, although they did not favour their application using gingival irrigators and recommended against the continual use of antiseptics in order to avoid the selection of resistant microorganisms [47]. Paradoxically, in their protocols on the prevention of IE secondary to dental manipulations published in 2004, the ESC and the BCS jointly with the RCP made no reference to the use of antiseptics before starting a manipulation [55,56].

In 2006, the BSAC recommended that, when possible, and in addition to the antibiotic prophylaxis, a pre-operative mouthrinse with 0.2% chlorhexidine gluconate should be performed, holding the antiseptic in the mouth for 1 minute [53]. In contrast, in its latest IE guideline, the Expert Committee of the AHA did not recommend the use of antiseptic prophylaxis before at-risk dental procedures [48].

With regard to the effect of chlorhexidine prophylaxis on the intensity and duration of bacteraemia following dental procedures, the NICE concluded that "*Chlorhexidine used as an oral rinse does not significantly reduce the level of bacteraemia following dental procedures*" [57]. This conclusion was reached after analysis of certain studies on the efficacy of chlorhexidine prophylaxis for the prevention of post-dental manipulation bacteraemia; those studies presented methodological differences with respect to the dental procedure performed, the concentration of chlorhexidine used, and the technique for applying the antiseptic solution (mouthwash and/or irrigation). These important differences make a comparison of the results between the different series inappropriate [59].

Very few studies have been published on the efficacy of mouth rinsing with 0.2% chlorhexidine (recommended by the BSAC in 2006) for the prevention of post-dental extraction bacteraemia [65]. Our research group demonstrated that initial rinsing with 0.2% chlorhexidine significantly reduced the duration of post-dental extraction bacteraemia [66,67]. These results allow us to speculate that the efficacy of antibiotic prophylaxis could be improved by the simultaneous application of chlorhexidine prophylaxis, although there is no scientific evidence to support this hypothesis.

The conclusions reached by the NICE on the lack of efficacy of antiseptic prophylaxis for the prevention of bacteraemia following dental procedures are based on a small volume of published scientific evidence [59]. At the present time, the controversies concerning the risk of developing IE of oral origin, the clinical repercussions of bacteraemia of oral origin, the efficacy of antibiotic prophylaxis and the risk-benefit and cost-benefit relationships of antibiotic prophylaxis could justify the reappraisal of the need for antibiotic prophylaxis for the prevention of IE currently being undertaken by the scientific community. Further research should be encouraged to confirm the efficacy of the recommended chlorhexidine regimens and to investigate new antiseptic protocols [59].

4. Conclusions

Over the past 50 years, prophylactic regimens for the prevention of IE secondary to dental procedures have been modified but remain consensus based. The indication for prophylaxis is now limited to patients with the highest risk of IE undergoing the highest risk dental procedures. The most recent prophylactic protocols published by the BSAC, the AHA and the ESC continue to recommend amoxicillin as the antibiotic of choice for oral prophylaxis. For individuals who are allergic to penicillins, the use of clindamycin, cephalexin or another first-generation oral cephalosporin, azithromycin or clarithromycin is recommended. However, the NICE has adopted a drastic stance in this respect, recommending the cessation of antibiotic prophylaxis for IE in individuals undergoing dental procedures in the United Kingdom. Further research should be encouraged to determine the impact of this recommendation of the NICE guideline.

All Expert Committees on IE prevention agree on the premise that "Good oral hygiene and regular dental checkups are of particular importance for the prevention of IE of oral origin".

Acknowledgements

This work was supported by project FIS 2011/PF004 (ref. PI11/01383) from the "Carlos III" Institute of Health, Madrid, Spain.

Author details

Inmaculada Tomás[1*] and Maximiliano Álvarez-Fernández[2]

*Address all correspondence to: inmaculada.tomas@usc.es

1 School of Medicine and Dentistry, Santiago de Compostela University, Spain

2 Xeral-Cies Hospital, Vigo, Spain

References

[1] Carmona, I. T, Diz-dios, P, & Scully, C. An update on the controversies in bacterial endocarditis of oral origin. Oral Surgery, Oral Medicine, Oral Pathology, Oral Radiology, and Endodontics (2002)., 93, 660-670.

[2] Pallasch, T. J. Antibiotic prophylaxis: problems in paradise. Dental Clinics of North America (2003)., 47, 665-679.

[3] Seymour, R. A, Lowry, R, Whitworth, J. M, & Martin, M. V. Infective endocarditis, dentistry and antibiotic prophylaxis; time for a rethink?. British Dental Journal (2000)., 189, 610-616.

[4] Beck, J, García, R, Heiss, G, Vokonas, P. S, & Offenbacher, S. Periodontal disease and cardiovascular disease. Journal of Periodontology (1996)., 67, 1123-1137.

[5] Destefano, F, Anda, R. F, Kahn, H. S, Williamson, D. F, & Russell, C. M. Dental disease and risk of coronary heart disease. British Medical Journal (Clinical Research ed.) (1993)., 306, 688-691.

[6] Olsen, I. Update on bacteraemia related to dental procedures. Transfusion and Apheresis Science (2008)., 39, 173-178.

[7] Stein, J. M, Kuch, B, Conrads, G, Fickl, S, Chrobot, J, Schulz, S, Ocklenburg, C, & Smeets, R. Clinical periodontal and microbiologic parameters in patients with acute myocardial infarction. Journal of Periodontology (2009)., 80, 1581-1589.

[8] Monteiro, A. M, Jardini, M. A, Alves, S, Giampaoli, V, Aubin, E. C, Figueiredo-neto, A. M, & Gidlund, M. Cardiovascular disease parameters in periodontitis. Journal of Periodontology (2009)., 80, 378-388.

[9] Dietrich, T, Jimenez, M, Krall-kaye, E. A, Vokonas, P. S, & Garcia, R. I. Age-dependent associations between chronic periodontitis/edentulism and risk of coronary heart disease. Circulation (2008)., 117, 1668-1674.

[10] Gaetti-Jardim E JrMarcelino SL, Feitosa AC, Romito GA, Avila-Campos MJ. Quantitative detection of periodontopathic bacteria in atherosclerotic plaques from coronary arteries. Journal of Medical Microbiology (2009)., 58, 1568-1575.

[11] Nakano, K, Nemoto, H, Nomura, R, Inaba, H, Yoshioka, H, Taniguchi, K, Amano, A, & Ooshima, T. Detection of oral bacteria in cardiovascular specimens. Oral Microbiology and Immunology (2009)., 24, 64-68.

[12] Pucar, A, Milasin, J, Lekovic, V, Vukadinovic, M, Ristic, M, Putnik, M, & Kenney, E. B. Correlation between atherosclerosis and periodontal putative pathogenic bacterial infections in coronary and internal mammary arteries. Journal of Periodontology (2007)., 78, 677-682.

[13] Okell, C. C, & Elliott, S. D. Bacteremia and oral sepsis with special reference to the aetiology of subacute endocarditis. Lancet (1935). , 2, 869-872.

[14] Burket, L. W, & Burn, C. G. Bacteremias following dental extraction. Demonstration of source of bacteria by means of a non-pathogen (*Serratia marcescens*). Journal of Dental Research (1937). , 16, 521-530.

[15] Palmer, H. R, & Kempf, M. *Streptococcus viridans* bacteremia following extraction of teeth; a case of multiple mycotic aneurysms in the pulmonary arteries: report of cases and necropsies. Journal of American Medical Association (1939). , 113, 1788-1792.

[16] Hopkins, J. A. *Streptococcus viridans*: bacteremia following extraction of the teeth. Journal of American Dental Association (1939). , 26, 2002-2008.

[17] Bender, I. B, & Pressman, R. S. Factors in dental bacteremia. Journal of American Dental Association (1945). , 32, 836-853.

[18] Rhoads, P. S, Schram, W. R, & Adair, D. Bacteremia following tooth extraction: prevention with penicillin and UN 445. Journal of American Dental Association (1950). , 41, 55-61.

[19] Robinson, L, Kraus, F. W, Lazansky, J. P, Wheeler, R. E, Gordon, S, & Johnson, V. Bacteremias of dental origin. II. A study of the factors influencing occurrence and detection. Oral Surgery (1950). , 3, 923-926.

[20] Brown, H. H. Tooth extraction and chronic infective endocarditis. Bristish Medical Journal (1932). , 1, 796-797.

[21] Abrahamson, L. Subacute bacterial endocarditis following removal of septic foci. British Medical Journal (1931). , 2, 8-9.

[22] Feldman, L, & Trace, I. M. Subacute bacterial endocarditis following removal of teeth or tonsils. Annals of Internal Medicine (1938). , 11, 2124-2132.

[23] Elliott, S. D. Bacteremia and oral sepsis. Proceedings of the Royal Society of Medicine (1939). , 32, 747-754.

[24] Fish, E. W, & Maclean, I. The distribution of oral streptococci in the tissues. British Dental Journal (1936). , 61, 336-362.

[25] Thomas, C. B, France, R, & Reichsman, F. Prophylactic use of sulfanilamide. Journal of American Medical Association (1941). , 116, 551-560.

[26] Hupp, J. R. Changing methods of preventing infective endocarditis following dental procedures: 1943-1993. Journal of Oral and Maxillofacial Surgery (1993). , 51, 616-623.

[27] Long, P. H, & Bliss, E. A. Clinical use of sulfanilamide, sulfapyridine and allied compounds. New York: MacMillan Co.; (1939).

[28] Kolmer, J. A, & Tuft, L. Clinical immunology, biotherapy and chemotherapy. Philadelphia: WB Saunders Co.; (1941).

[29] Spink, W. W. Sulfanilamide and related compounds in general practice. Chicago: Year Book Publishers; (1941).

[30] Budnitz, E, Nizel, A. E, & Berg, L. Prophylactic use of sulfapyridine in patients susceptible to subacute bacterial endocarditis following dental surgical procedures. Preliminary report. Journal of American Dental Association (1942)., 29, 346-349.

[31] Northrop, P. M, & Crowley, M. C. The prophylactic use of sulfathiazole in transient bacteremia following the extraction of teeth. Journal of Oral Surgery (1943)., 1, 19-29.

[32] Northrop, P. M, & Crowley, M. C. Further studies on the effect of the prophylactic use of sulfathiazole and sulfamerazine on bacteremia following extraction of teeth. Journal of Oral Surgery (1944)., 2, 134-140.

[33] Hirsh, H. L, Vivino, J. J, Merril, A, & Dowling, H. F. Effect of prophylactically administered penicillin on incidence of bacteremia following extraction of teeth. Archives of Internal Medicine (1948)., 81, 868-878.

[34] Glaser, R. J, Dankner, A, Mathes, S. B, & Harford, C. G. Effect of penicillin on the bacteremia following dental extraction. American Journal of Medicine (1948)., 4, 55-65.

[35] Rhoads, P. S, & Schram, W. R. Bacteremia following tooth extraction; prevention with penicillin and dimethyl-5-sulfanilamide-isoxazole (Gantrosan). Proceedings of Twenty-first Annual Meeting. Journal of Laboratory and Clinical Medicine (1948)., 3, 4.

[36] Thoma, K. H. Oral Surgery. St Louis: Mosby Co.; (1948).

[37] Archer, W. H. A manual of oral surgery. Philadelphia: Saunders Co.; (1952).

[38] Mead, S. V. Oral surgery. St Louis: Mosby Co.; (1954).

[39] American Heart AssociationPrevention of rheumatic fever and bacterial endocarditis through control of streptococcal infections. Circulation (1955)., 11, 317-320.

[40] Tomás Carmona IDiz Dios P, Scully C. Efficacy of antibiotic prophylactic regimens for the prevention of bacterial endocarditis of oral origin. Journal of Dental Research (2007)., 86, 1142-1159.

[41] American Heart AssociationPrevention of rheumatic fever and bacterial endocarditis through control of streptococcal infections. Circulation (1960)., 21, 151-155.

[42] Wannamaker, L. W, Denny, F. W, Diehl, A, & Jawetz, E. Kirby WMM, Markowitz M, McCarty M, Mortimer EA, Paterson PY, Perry W, Rammelkamp CH Jr, Stollerman GH (Committee on Prevention of Rheumatic Fever and Bacterial Endocarditis, American Heart Association). Prevention of bacterial endocarditis. Circulation (1965)., 31, 953-954.

[43] American Heart AssociationPrevention of bacterial endocarditis. Journal of American Dental Association (1972)., 85, 1377-1379.

[44] Kaplan, E. L, Anthony, B. F, Bisno, A, Durack, D, Houser, H, Millard, H. D, Sanford, J, Shulman, S. T, Stollerman, M, & Taranta, A. Wenger N (Committee on Rheumatic Fever and Bacterial Endocarditis, American Heart Association). Prevention of bacterial endocarditis. Circulation (1977). A-143A.

[45] Shulman, S. T, Amren, D. P, Bisno, A. L, Dajani, A. S, Durack, D. T, Gerber, M. A, Kaplan, E. L, Millard, H. D, Sanders, W. E, & Schwartz, R. H. Watanakunakorn C (Committee on Rheumatic Fever and Infective Endocarditis, American Heart Association). Prevention of bacterial endocarditis: a statement for health professionals by the Committee on cardiovascular disease in the young. Circulation (1984). A-1127A.

[46] Dajani, A. S, Bisno, A. L, Chung, K. J, Durack, D. T, Freed, M, Gerber, M. A, Karchmer, A. W, Millard, H. D, Rahimtoola, S, Shulman, S. T, Watanakunakorn, C, & Taubert, K. A. Prevention of bacterial endocarditis: recommendations by the American Heart Association. Journal of American Medical Association (1990). , 264, 2919-2922.

[47] Dajani, A. S, Taubert, K. A, Wilson, W, Bolger, A. F, Bayer, A, Ferrieri, P, Gewitz, M. H, Shulman, S. T, Nouri, S, Newburger, J. W, Hutto, C, Pallasch, T. J, Gage, T. W, Levison, M. E, & Peter, G. Zuccaro G Jr. Prevention of bacterial endocarditis: recommendations by the American Heart Association. Journal of American Medical Association (1997). , 277, 1794-1801.

[48] Wilson, W, Taubert, K. A, Gewitz, M, Lockhart, P. B, Baddour, L. M, Levison, M, Bolger, A, Cabell, C. H, Takahashi, M, Baltimore, R. S, Newburger, J. W, Strom, B. L, Tani, L. Y, Gerber, M, Bonow, R. O, Pallasch, T, Shulman, S. T, Rowley, A. H, Burns, J. C, Ferrieri, P, Gardner, T, Goff, D, & Durack, D. T. Prevention of infective endocarditis: guidelines from the American Heart Association. Circulation (2007). , 116, 1736-1754.

[49] [No authors listed]The antibiotic prophylaxis of infective endocarditis: report of a working party of the British Society for Antimicrobial Chemotherapy. Lancet (1982). , 11, 1323-1326.

[50] Simmons, N. A, Cawson, R. A, Clarke, C. A, Eykyn, S. J, Geddes, A. M, Littler, W. A, Mcgowan, D. A, Oakley, C. M, & Shanson, D. C. Prophylaxis of infective endocarditis. Lancet (1986).

[51] [No authors listed]Antibiotic prophylaxis of infective endocarditis: recommendations from the endocarditis working party of the British Society for Antimicrobial Chemotherapy. Lancet (1990). , 13, 88-89.

[52] Simmons, N. A, Ball, A. P, Cawson, R. A, Eykyn, S. J, Littler, W. A, Mcgowan, D. A, Oakley, C. M, & Shanson, D. C. Antibiotic prophylaxis and infective endocarditis. Lancet (1992). , 339, 1292-1293.

[53] Gould, F. K, Elliot, T. S, Foweraker, J, Fulford, M, Perry, J. D, Roberts, G. J, Sandoe, J. A, & Watkin, R. W. Working Party of the British Society for Antimicrobial Chemotherapy. Guidelines for the prevention of endocarditis: report of the Working Party

of the British Society for Antimicrobial Chemotherapy. Journal of Antimicrobial Chemotherapy (2006). , 57, 1035-1042.

[54] Leport, C, Horstkotte, D, & Burckhardt, D. and the group of experts of the International Society for Chemotherapy. European Heart Journal (1995). suppl. B):, 126-131.

[55] Horstkotte, D, Follath, F, Gutschik, E, Lengyel, M, Oto, A, Pavie, A, Soler-soler, J, Thiene, G, Von Graevenitz, A, Priori, S. G, Garcia, M. A, Blanc, J. J, Budaj, A, Cowie, M, Dean, V, & Deckers, J. Fernández Burgos E, Lekakis J, Lindahl B, Mazzotta G, Morais J, Oto A, Smiseth OA, Lekakis J, Vahanian A, Delahaye F, Parkhomenko A, Filipatos G, Aldershvile J, Vardas P; Task Force Members on Infective Endocarditis of the European Society of Cardiology; ESC Committee for Practice Guidelines (CPG); Document Reviewers. Guidelines on prevention, diagnosis and treatment of infective endocarditis executive summary: the task force on infective endocarditis of the European Society of Cardiology. European Heart Journal (2004). , 25, 267-276.

[56] Dental aspects of endocarditis prophylaxis: new recommendations from a working group of the Bristish Cardiac Society Clinical Practice Committee and Royal College of Physicians Clinical Effectiveness and Evaluation; (2004). http://www.bcs.com/library.accessed June 2012].

[57] National Institute for Health and Clinical ExcellenceProphylaxis against infective endocarditis. United Kingdom [WWW document]; 2008. http://www.nice.org.uk/nicemedia/pdf/PIEGuidelines.pdf.accessed June (2012).

[58] Task Force on the PreventionDiagnosis, and Treatment of Infective Endocarditis of the European Society of Cardiology; European Society of Clinical Microbiology and Infectious Diseases; International Society of Chemotherapy for Infection and Cancer, Habib G, Hoen B, Tornos P, Thuny F, Prendergast B, Vilacosta I, Moreillon P, of Jesus Antunes M, Thilen U, Lekakis J, Lengyel M, Müller L, Naber CK, Nihoyannopoulos P, Moritz A, Zamorano JL; ESC Committee for Practice Guidelines, Vahanian A, Auricchio A, Bax J, Ceconi C, Dean V, Filippatos G, Funck-Brentano C, Hobbs R, Kearney P, McDonagh T, McGregor K, Popescu BA, Reiner Z, Sechtem U, Sirnes PA, Tendera M, Vardas P, Widimsky P. Guidelines on the prevention, diagnosis, and treatment of infective endocarditis (new version 2009): the Task Force on the Prevention, Diagnosis, and Treatment of Infective Endocarditis of the European Society of Cardiology (ESC). European Heart Journal (2009). , 30, 2369-2413.

[59] Tomás, I, Limeres, J, & Diz, P. Confirm the efficacy. British Dental Journal (2008).

[60] Thornhill, M. H, Dayer, M. J, Forde, J. M, Corey, G. R, Hock, G, Chu, V. H, Couper, D. J, & Lockhart, P. B. Impact of the NICE guideline recommending cessation of antibiotic prophylaxis for prevention of infective endocarditis: before and after study. British Medical Journal (2011). d2392.

[61] Schweizerischen Arbeitsgruppe fur Endokarditisprophylaxe: prophylaxe der bakteriellen endokarditisSchweizerische Medizinische Wochenschrift (1984). , 114, 1146-1152.

[62] Diz Dios PTomás Carmona I, Limeres Posse J, Medina Hernández J, Fernández Feijoo J, Álvaréz Fernández M. Comparative efficacies of amoxicillin, clindamycin, and moxifloxacin in prevention of bacteremia following dental extractions. Antimicrobial Agents and Chemotherapy (2006). , 50, 2996-3002.

[63] Shanson, D. New British and American guidelines for the antibiotic prophylaxis of infective endocarditis: do the changes make sense?. A critical review. Current Opinion in Infectious Diseases (2008). , 21, 191-199.

[64] Duval, X, & Leport, C. Prophylaxis of infective endocarditis: current tendencies, continuing controversies. Lancet Infectious Diseases (2008). , 8, 225-232.

[65] Lockhart, P. B. An analysis of bacteremias during dental extractions. A double-blind, placebo-controlled study of chlorhexidine. Archives of Internal Medicine (1996). , 156, 513-520.

[66] Tomás, I, Álvarez, M, Limeres, J, Tomás, M, Medina, J, Otero, J. L, & Diz, P. Effect of chlorhexidine mouthwash on the risk of post-extraction bacteremia. Infection Control and Hospital Epidemiology (2007). , 28, 577-582.

[67] Diz, P. Tomás Carmona I, Barbosa M, Amaral B, Cerqueira C, Limeres J, Álvarez M. A chlorhexidine mouthwash reduces the risk of bacteraemia following dental extractions performed under either general or local anaesthesia. Clinical Research in Cardiology (2007). , 96, 443-444.

Chapter 5

Surgical Management of Infective Endocarditis

Nicholas Kang and Warren Smith

Additional information is available at the end of the chapter

http://dx.doi.org/10.5772/56761

1. Introduction

'The advent of a wide spectrum of bactericidal antibiotic agents has enabled physicians to treat many cases of bacterial endocarditis with a high likelihood of success. There remain, however, a significant number of patients with endocarditis in whom the infection is more resistant to antimicrobial therapy, valve destruction more rapid, and a satisfactory response to medical therapy sufficiently infrequent to warrant consideration of a new therapeutic approach'.

Circulation 1965;13:450.

Thus began the first published case report of cardiac valve replacement for infective endocarditis by Doctors Wallace, Young and Osterhout of Duke University Medical Centre. They described a 45 year old man with Klebsiella endocarditis affecting the aortic valve in whom severe aortic regurgitation and congestive heart failure developed which failed to respond to medical therapy. Excision of the valve and replacement with a Starr-Edwards prosthesis was curative. [1]

In fact, the first surgical attempts to treat infective endocarditis date back to 1937, prior to the introduction of antibiotics, when John Strieder at the Massachusetts Memorial Hospital in Boston ligated an infected ductus arteriosus. The patient was a 22-year old female in grave condition. It was a matter of controversy whether ductus ligation would heal endocarditis or, on the contrary, perhaps even exacerbate it. [2] The surgery proved difficult, and although the patient's immediate postoperative condition was excellent, with the typical sound of an open ductus no longer heard, she died four days later. Postmortem examination revealed vegetations extending from the origin of the ductus to the pulmonary valve.

Over the ensuing decades, developments in open-heart surgery and the evolution of cardiac valvular prostheses have since made surgery for endocarditis part of the routine work of every cardiac surgical unit. Nevertheless, such surgery still poses unique challenges and carries substantial risk of morbidity and mortality. Furthermore, the indications, timing, and type of surgery remain controversial as there are few randomized trials to guide patient management.

2. Surgical anatomy of the heart valves

It is important to appreciate that the four cardiac valves do not exist in isolation, but are closely related to each other and also to other vital intracardiac structures. [Figure 1]

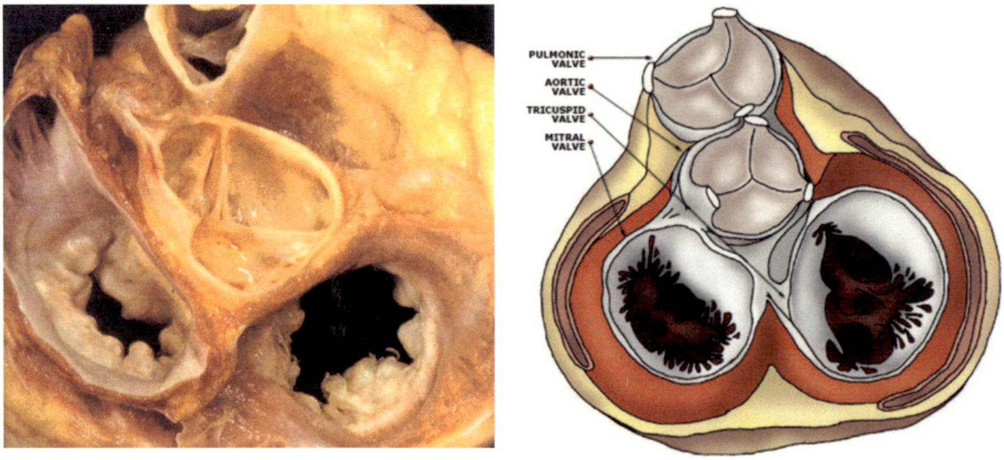

Figure 1. The four cardiac valves. Note the central position of the aortic valve and the fibrous skeleton of the heart connecting mitral, tricuspid and aortic valves. Reproduced from reference [3]

The aortic, mitral and tricuspid valves are all connected at the membranous septum [4], a small but crucial part of the heart [see Figure 2]. It separates the left ventricle from the right ventricle (interventricular component), and also separates the left ventricle from the right atrium (atrioventricular component). The conduction tissue (penetrating bundle) is intimately related to the membranous septum, being sandwiched between it and the muscular septum. [3] Only the pulmonary valve lacks fibrous continuity with the other valves, being situated on a circumferential sleeve of cardiac muscle known as the infundibulum.

It can therefore be appreciated how a virulent, invasive intracardiac infection might become potentially so destructive. Not only can the primary valve be affected, but infection can spread into adjacent valves, fistulas can develop into the cardiac chambers or pericardial space, the fibrous skeleton of the heart can be eroded and the conduction system can be destroyed.

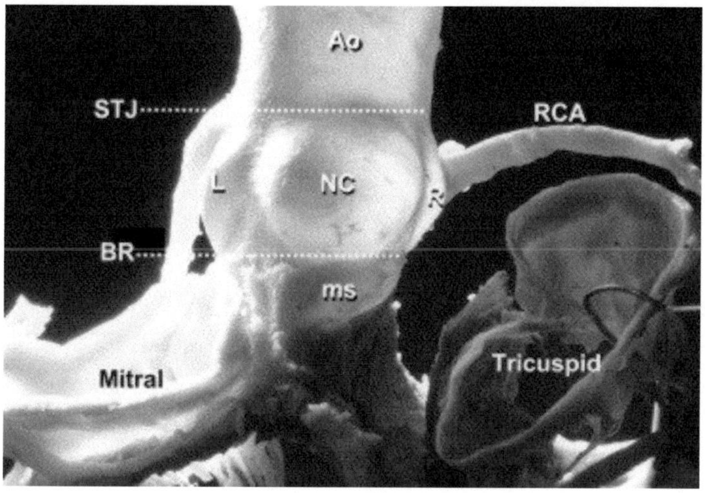

Figure 2. Membranous septum. The tricuspid annulus has been detached from the membranous septum in this prosection. Ao aorta, BR basal ring, L left coronary sinus, ms membranous septum, NC non coronary sinus, RCA right coronary artery, STJ sinotubular junction. Reproduced with permission from reference [4]

3. Indications for surgery in native valve endocarditis

The proportion of patients with endocarditis treated surgically varies widely amongst individual units, reflecting the fact that most indications for surgery are not absolute. Large multicentre studies report overall rates of surgery of approximately 40-50%. [5-7]

In recent years, international guidelines for valvular heart surgery and, more specifically, infective endocarditis have been published by a number of collaborative task forces. These task forces have examined the relevant scientific literature available and made evidence based recommendations accordingly for best practice guidelines.

The American College of Cardiology and American Heart Association (ACC/AHA) published their updated guidelines for valvular heart disease in 2008. [8] A section of these guidelines is devoted to infective endocarditis. In native valve endocarditis (NVE), the strongest recommendations for surgery apply to those patients with signs of heart failure, adverse haemodynamic effects from regurgitant valve lesions, antibiotic resistant organisms, or locally invasive cardiac infection with destruction of perivalvular structures. The recommendation for surgery is present, but weaker, in patients with recurrent embolic events and/or very large vegetations. Table 1 summarises these recommendations.

Class I
1. Surgery of the native valve is indicated in patients with acute infective endocarditis who present with valve stenosis or regurgitation resulting in heart failure. *(Level of Evidence: B)* 2. Surgery of the native valve is indicated in patients with acute infective endocarditis who present with AR or MR with hemodynamic evidence of elevated LV end-diastolic or left atrial pressures (e.g., premature closure of MV with AR, rapid decelerating MR signal by continuous wave Doppler (v-wave cutoff sign), or moderate or severe pulmonary hypertension). *(Level of Evidence: B)* 3. Surgery of the native valve is indicated in patients with infective endocarditis caused by fungal or other highly resistant organisms. *(Level of Evidence: B)* 4. Surgery of the native valve is indicated in patients with infective endocarditis complicated by heart block, annular or aortic abscess, or destructive penetrating lesions (e.g., sinus of Valsalva to right atrium, right ventricle, or left atrium fistula; mitral leaflet perforation with aortic valve endocarditis; or infection in annulus fibrosa). *(Level of Evidence: B)*
Class IIa
1. Surgery of the native valve is reasonable in patients with infective endocarditis who present with recurrent emboli and persistent vegetations despite appropriate antibiotic therapy. *(Level of Evidence: C)*
Class IIb
1. Surgery of the native valve may be considered in patients with infective endocarditis who present with mobile vegetations in excess of 10 mm with or without emboli. *(Level of Evidence: C)*

Class I: Conditions for which there is evidence for and/or general agreement that the procedure or treatment is beneficial, useful, and effective.

Class II: Conditions for which there is conflicting evidence and/or a divergence of opinion about the usefulness/efficacy of a procedure or treatment.

Class IIa: Weight of evidence/opinion is in favor of usefulness/efficacy.

Class IIb: Usefulness/efficacy is less well established by evidence/opinion.

Class III: Conditions for which there is evidence and/or general agreement that the procedure/treatment is not useful/effective and in some cases may be harmful. In addition, the weight of evidence in support of the recommendation is listed as follows:

- Level of Evidence A: Data derived from multiple randomized clinical trials.
- Level of Evidence B: Data derived from a single randomized trial or nonrandomized studies.
- Level of Evidence C: Only consensus opinion of experts, case studies, or standard-of-care.

Table 1. AHA/ACC guidelines for NVE

The ACC/AHA guidelines also state that "prosthetic valve endocarditis and native valve endocarditis caused by Staphylococcus aureus are almost always surgical diseases", suggesting that this organism causes particularly virulent intracardiac infection which tends to be more destructive and consequently more difficult to eradicate with antibiotic treatment alone.

http://dx.doi.org/10.5772/56761

In 2009, the European Society of Cardiology (ESC) published their own set of guidelines on the prevention, diagnosis and treatment of endocarditis. [9] The recommendations for surgery follow similar themes to the ACC/AHA guidelines, with heart failure, uncontrolled infection and prevention of embolism representing the three broad categories of indications for surgery (see Table 2).

Indications for surgery in NVE	**Timing**	**Class**	**Level**
A – HEART FAILURE			
Aortic or mitral IE with severe acute regurgitation or valve obstruction causing refractory pulmonary oedema or cardiogenic shock	Emergency	I	B
Aortic or mitral IE with fistula into a cardiac chamber or pericardium causing refractory pulmonary oedema or cardiogenic shock	Emergency	I	B
Aortic or mitral IE with severe acute regurgitation or valve obstruction and persisting heart failure or echocardiographic signs of poor haemodynamic tolerance (early mitral closure or pulmonary hypertension)	Urgent	I	B
Aortic or mitral IE with severe regurgitation and no HF	Elective	IIa	B
B-UNCONTROLLED INFECTION			
Locally uncontrolled infection (abscess, false aneurysm, fistula, enlarging vegetation)	Urgent	I	B
Persisting fever and positive blood cultures >7-10 days	Urgent	I	B
Infection caused by fungi or multiresistant organisms	Urgent/elective	I	B
C- PREVENTION OF EMBOLISM			
Aortic or mitral IE with large vegetations (>10mm) following one or more embolic episodes despite appropriate antibiotic therapy	Urgent	I	B
Aortic or mitral IE with large vegetations (>10mm) and other predictors of complicated course (heart failure, persistent infection, abscess)	Urgent	I	C
Isolated very large vegetations (>15mm)	urgent	IIb	C

Table 2. ESC guidelines for NVE

More recently published data from a large non-randomised prospective multicentre trial of 1552 patients with NVE found an overall survival benefit for surgery compared with medical therapy (12.1% mortality versus 20.7%). [10] In subgroup analysis using propensity scores, surgery was found to confer a survival benefit compared with medical therapy among patients with a higher propensity for surgery and those with paravalvular complications, systemic embolization, Staphylococcus aureus NVE and stroke.

Surprisingly, neither valve perforation nor congestive heart failure predicted a survival benefit for early surgery in this study, which goes against prior assumptions and experiences. [11] It may be that the severity of heart failure, which was not specified in the study, does in fact influence outcome as reported by others. [12]

4. Timing of surgery

Deciding upon the optimal timing of surgery is one of the great difficulties in managing patients with endocarditis. As Farzaneh-Far and Bolger state in a recent editorial, "the decision to commit to a surgical procedure that might possibly be avoided is quite difficult for the patient, the surgeon, and the referring physician...Because patients with endocarditis span such a wide range of comorbidities, complications, and manifestations, generalization from a disparate population is unsatisfying." [11]

The difficulty is compounded by the fact that available evidence to recommend timing of surgery in endocarditis is largely limited to observational data and expert opinion. Studies employing propensity modelling to try and overcome selection bias have been reported. [10] More recently, the first randomized controlled trial in endocarditis was published to help define the optimal timing of surgery, [13] as discussed below.

The timing of surgery can be considered in the following clinical situations:

a. Congestive heart failure.

The ESC guidelines advise emergency surgery for patients with persistent pulmonary oedema or cardiogenic shock, and urgent surgery when heart failure is less severe. [9] In patients with well tolerated severe valvular insufficiency (i.e. mild or no heart failure) and no other reasons for surgery, the guidelines recommend 'medical management with antibiotics under strict clinical and echocardiographic observation' with surgery to be considered 'after healing of infective endocarditis, depending on tolerance of the valve lesion'.

b. Systemic embolism

Systemic embolism occurs in up to 50% of patients with infective endocarditis, most frequently to the central nervous system and specifically to the territory of the middle cerebral artery [14]. A number of studies have demonstrated that embolic risk falls substantially after the first 2-3 weeks of treatment. [15, 16] The presence of large (>15mm on echocardiogram) vegetations has been considered a relative indication for early surgery, particularly in Staphylococcal endocarditis affecting the mitral valve. [15]

Recently the benefit of early surgery in this context was investigated in the first randomized trial in endocarditis [13]. In this study, 76 patients with left-sided native valve infective endocarditis, vegetations greater than 10 mm, and severe valve dysfunction were randomly assigned to surgery within 48 hours or antibiotic therapy. The primary end point was a composite of embolic events or death within 6 weeks after randomization. Secondary end points were embolic events, recurrent endocarditis, repeat hospitalization due to the development of congestive heart failure, or death from any cause at 6 months.

The major finding in this study was that early surgery significantly reduced the composite end point of embolic events and death from any cause, by effectively decreasing the risk of systemic embolism. The authors suggest that early surgery is therefore a valuable therapeutic option to prevent embolism.

c. Embolic stroke

Timing of surgery after embolic stroke poses an especially difficult dilemma. Early surgery carries a risk of haemorrhagic transformation of cerebral infarction, whilst delaying surgery may lead to further embolic events and/or worsening of cardiac function. In a recent review of 100 published studies, Rossi et al concluded that "evidence is conflicting because of lack of controlled studies" [17]. They state that "the optimal timing for the valve replacement depends on the type of neurological complication and the urgency of the operation."

The ESC guidelines suggest that if cerebral haemorrhage has been excluded and neurological damage is not severe, surgery should not be delayed. [9] The risk of further neurological complication is low and full neurological recovery may be possible.

Conversely, in cases with intracranial haemorrhage, neurological prognosis is worse and ESC guidelines suggest that surgery should be postponed for at least one month. If the possibility of mycotic aneurysm is suspected, the patient should be evaluated with cerebral angiography as such aneurysms are a contraindication for anticoagulation as well. [18]

In all such cases, consultation with neurology and neurosurgical teams is advisable.

d. Paravalvular extension

As emphasized in the preceding section on cardiac anatomy, paravalvular abscess formation has a high probability of impairing cardiac conduction and leading to multi-valve involvement. Extension of infection is very common in prosthetic valve endocarditis and affects 10-40% of native aortic valve infection. The diagnosis is best made by transoesophageal echocardiography and should be suspected whenever there is any degree of atrioventricular block present. Urgent surgery is indicated once the diagnosis is made.

5. Decision making

It is evident from the above that decision making with regards to both the indications and timing of surgery is still problematic. Because infective endocarditis can have such variable clinical manifestations, treatment must of necessity be tailored to individual patient circumstances, the nature of the organism, its effect on the heart and other organs, duration of antibiotic therapy already received, progression of disease over time, and numerous other considerations.

Currently available guidelines aid decision making but are founded largely on observational data. Despite the protean difficulties in designing randomized trials in endocarditis, the pioneering study cited above [13] illustrates that the task is not impossible. Given that endocarditis remains a frequent, important and potentially lethal condition, the challenge of acquiring more definitive evidence should be accepted.

6. Operative management

Surgery for endocarditis can be amongst the most challenging operations faced by the cardiac surgeon. Debriding infected cardiac tissue and restoring anatomical and functional integrity can be a test of considerable surgical skill. Furthermore, patients present for operation in varying degrees of septicaemia, cardiac failure, multiorgan failure, shock, coagulopathy, hypoproteinemia and anasarca, to which the further insults of surgical trauma and cardiopulmonary bypass are added.

6.1. Surgical principles

The primary objectives of surgery are (1) eradication of all infected, necrotic and non-viable tissue and (2) reconstruction of cardiac morphology. [9] How this is achieved surgically is very dependent upon the local extent of intracardiac infection. Surgery may thus entail repair or replacement of one or more valves, complete aortic root replacement, debridement and patching of abscesses, closure of fistulas, or reconstruction of part of the fibrous skeleton of the heart. Cardiac transplantation has even been reported in an extreme case of relapsing 'burnt out' endocarditis with multiple previous unsuccessful surgeries over many years. [19]

6.2. Valve repair

Valve repair, rather than replacement, is theoretically an attractive option in endocarditis when infection is limited in its local extent. Not only does repair avoid the inherent problems of prosthetic valves (e.g. anticoagulation, thromboembolism, paravalvular leak, structural valve deterioration) but it reduces the risk of recurrent endocarditis when compared with valve replacement. [20].

Techniques may involve simple vegetectomy alone, patching of leaflet perforations with pericardium, or more sophisticated methods of leaflet and/or chordal reconstruction. The method used must be tailored to the individual pathology present (see Figure 4). Eradicating the infection and achieving a durably competent valve is the goal of repair.

Valve repair techniques are now well established for the treatment of degenerative mitral valve disease, but are not always feasible in the setting of endocarditis. In a metanalysis of 24 studies comparing repair versus replacement in 1194 patients, 39% of patients underwent repair whilst the remainder required replacement. Repair was associated with superior early and late outcomes, with reduced need for repeat mitral surgery, fewer cerebrovascular events and fewer episodes of recurrent endocarditis. Operative mortality was less than 10% and 5-year survival greater than 80%. [20]

It is important to appreciate, however, that all 24 studies in the metanalysis were retrospective observational series and thus subject to both selection bias and publication bias. As was noted

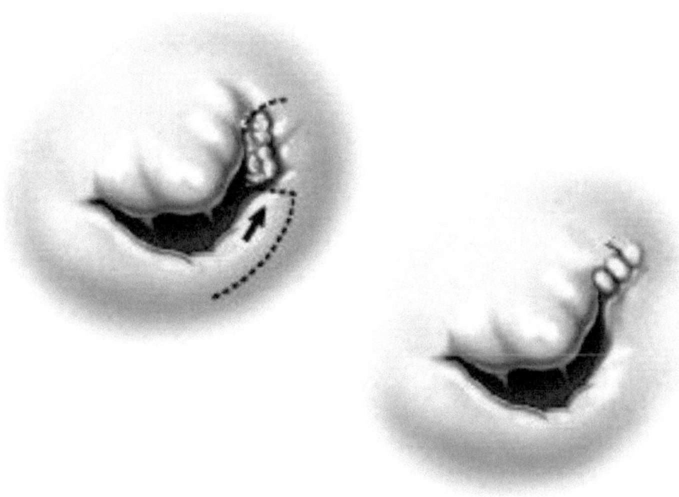

Figure 3. Mitral valve repair. Reproduced with permission from reference [21]. The vegetation involving the posteromedial commissure has been resected, and the posterior leaflet mobilised and advanced into the commissure. The valve must be competent following repair, otherwise replacement will be necessary.

in the meta-analysis, "the validity of comparing mitral valve repair with mitral valve replacement may be questioned. Mitral valve replacement is often reserved for the sickest patients in whom mitral valve repair cannot be performed. Therefore, it would not be surprising that postoperative results would be worse for these patients." [20]

Valve repair is a much less well established but nonetheless emerging technique in aortic valve disease. Mayer et al reported a series of 100 patients undergoing surgery for aortic valve endocarditis; 33 treated by repair and 67 by replacement. [22] Five year survival was significantly higher in the repair group, although again this was a retrospective series with inherent selection bias. In addition, it is worth noting that the subgroup of patients with repaired bicuspid valves had a higher rate of late aortic regurgitation.

6.3. Valve replacement

Valve replacement, as first performed by Dr W Glenn Young Jr at the Duke University Medical Center [1] nearly 50 years ago, remains the standard of care in the majority of cases of endocarditis treated surgically.

The optimal choice of valve substitute in the setting of infective endocarditis has long been debated. Once again, only observational data rather than randomized clinical trials are available to guide clinical practice.

Some investigators have reported that valve replacement using a homograft results in a lower rate of recurrent endocarditis. [23, 24] Most surgeons now believe that the choice of valve substitute is less important in determining recurrence than the completeness of debridement at the time of operation. Homografts have the disadvantage of more difficult reoperation at the time of their inevitable structural deterioration. For NVE confined to the valve leaflets, operative results are similar for mechanical and biological prostheses. [25, 8]

6.4. Aortic root replacement

Sometimes, simple valve replacement may not be sufficient when dealing with paravalvular infection, resulting in reinfection of the prosthesis, valve dehiscence, or both. [18] This is often the case in prosthetic valve endocarditis (see below) Aortic root replacement, as opposed to simple aortic valve replacement, may therefore be necessary in these circumstances. Aortic root replacement involves excision of the aortic valve cusps, the sinuses of Valsalva, and a variable amount of the distal ascending aorta. The coronary arteries have to be reimplanted into the replaced root.

In these situations, root replacement with a homograft can be advantageous. The homograft aortic root is soft, pliable, and can be tailored to patch abscess cavities and rebuild tissue defects, especially if the anterior mitral leaflet of the homograft has been left attached. [24]

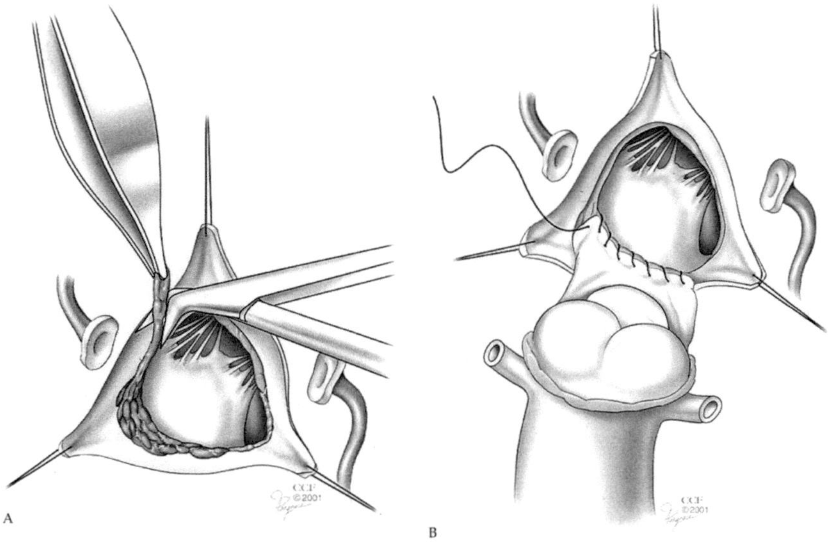

Figure 4. Aortic root replacement using a homograft. Reproduced with permission from reference [24]. The attached homograft mitral leaflet has been used to reconstruct the debrided abscess cavity in the aortic-mitral curtain

Homografts, however, are limited in their availability. Stentless xenograft valves exhibit similar properties to homografts and have been used in this setting as an alternative. [26] Standard mechanical valved conduits have also been used with very satisfactory results. [27, 28] The pulmonary autograft (Ross procedure) is another option although this adds greater complexity to an already difficult procedure in a sick patient. As previously emphasised, the completeness of debridement is probably more important than the type of cardiac replacement tissue used.

http://dx.doi.org/10.5772/56761

6.5. Reconstruction of the fibrous skeleton

In very advanced cases of endocarditis, there may be extensive tissue destruction around the aorto-ventricular junction, mitral annulus and aorto-mitral curtain. In addition to replacing both aortic and mitral valves, the fibrous skeleton of the heart itself may need to be reconstructed. (see Figure 5). Such patients may in fact prove to be beyond surgical repair and deemed inoperable. Complex techniques of surgical reconstruction have been reported by some groups, notably David et al. [29]

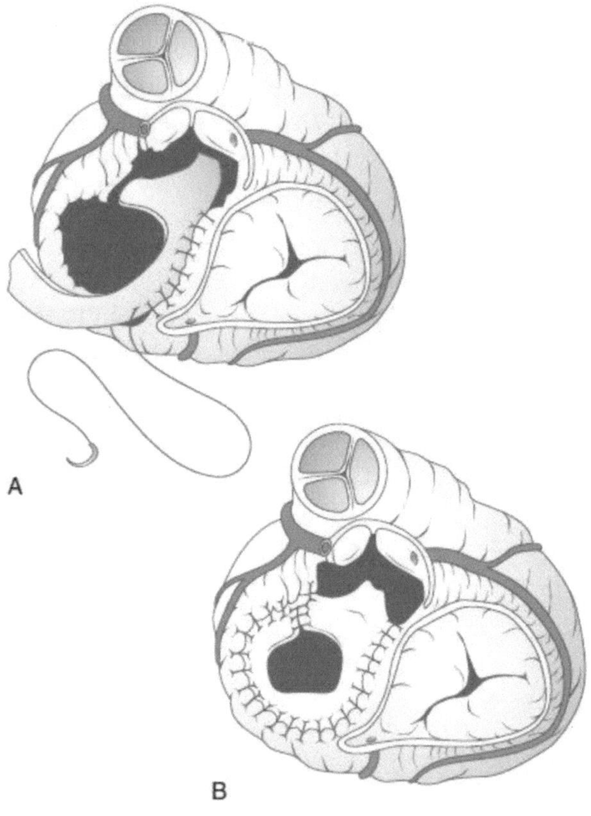

Figure 5. Complex reconstruction of the mitral annulus and aortic-mitral curtain using a pericardial patch. Reproduced with permission from reference [29]. Both aortic and mitral valves have been excised, as well as the intervening area of fibrous continuity (aortic-mitral curtain). The patch acts as a new fibrous skeleton upon which to anchor sutures to secure the aortic and mitral valve prostheses.

7. Prosthetic valve endocarditis

Prosthetic valve endocarditis (PVE) is one of the most feared conditions in cardiac surgery. It accounts for approximately 20% of cases of IE. [7] Mechanical and bioprosthetic valves are equally affected at a frequency in the order of 1% per patient year.

PVE is traditionally classified into early (within 60 days of original valve replacement surgery) and late (greater than 60 days), although a cut-off of 12 months has been suggested by some. [30] The implication is that in early PVE the infection has been acquired at the time of original surgery, whereas in late PVE it complicates a subsequent unrelated bacteraemic episode.

The rate of paravalvular infection is much higher in PVE than NVE, owing to the presence of the prosthetic sewing ring. With mechanical valve prostheses, paravalvular abscess is present in virtually all cases. With bioprosthetic valves, infection is sometimes confined to the valve leaflets, but more often the sewing ring is involved as well.

Paravalvular infection in the aortic position can rapidly lead to aortic root abscess, fistulas into cardiac chambers, disruption of the aortic-mitral curtain, and even complete aorto-ventricular dehiscence. [24, 26] Surgery to remedy these problems is made substantially more complex in view of the fact that these are reoperations. This degree of surgical complexity is reflected in the operative mortality, which is typically double that for NVE surgery [7, 31, 32] (see 'Results of Surgery' section below).

The decision as to whether to operate or not for PVE is difficult. Operative risk is much greater for PVE than NVE, but the mortality with medical treatment alone is similarly higher, resulting in a management dilemma. Essentially, patients with early PVE, Staphylococcal PVE and complicated PVE (abscess, heart failure, prosthetic valve dysfunction) are more likely to require surgery whereas late PVE, non-Staphylococcal PVE and uncomplicated PVE can be managed medically with close follow-up. [9]

Tables 3 and 4 summarise the AHA/ACC and ESC guidelines respectively for PVE.

Class I
1. Consultation with a cardiac surgeon is indicated for patients with infective endocarditis of a prosthetic valve. *(Level of Evidence: C)*
2. Surgery is indicated for patients with infective endocarditis of a prosthetic valve who present with heart failure. *(Level of Evidence: B)*
3. Surgery is indicated for patients with infective endocarditis of a prosthetic valve who present with dehiscence evidenced by cine fluoroscopy or echocardiography. *(Level of Evidence: B)*
4. Surgery is indicated for patients with infective endocarditis of a prosthetic valve who present with evidence of increasing obstruction or worsening regurgitation. *(Level of Evidence: C)*
5. Surgery is indicated for patients with infective endocarditis of a prosthetic valve who present with complications (e.g., abscess formation). *(Level of Evidence: C)*
Class IIa
1. Surgery is reasonable for patients with infective endocarditis of a prosthetic valve who present with evidence of persistent bacteremia or recurrent emboli despite appropriate antibiotic treatment. *(Level of Evidence: C)*
2. Surgery is reasonable for patients with infective endocarditis of a prosthetic valve who present with relapsing infection. *(Level of Evidence: C)*
Class III
1. Routine surgery is not indicated for patients with uncomplicated infective endocarditis of a prosthetic valve caused by first infection with a sensitive organism. *(Level of Evidence: C)*

Table 3. AHA/ACC guidelines for PVE

http://dx.doi.org/10.5772/56761

Indications for surgery in PVE	Timing	Class	Level
A – HEART FAILURE			
PVE with severe prosthetic dysfunction (dehiscence or obstruction) causing refractory pulmonary oedema or cardiogenic shock	Emergency	I	B
PVE with fistula into a cardiac chamber or pericardium causing refractory pulmonary oedema or cardiogenic shock	Emergency	I	B
PVE with severe prosthetic dysfunction and persisting heart failure	Urgent	I	B
Severe prosthetic dehiscence without HF	Elective	I	B
B-UNCONTROLLED INFECTION			
Locally uncontrolled infection (abscess, false aneurysm, fistula, enlarging vegetation)	Urgent	I	B
PVE caused by fungi or multiresistant organisms	Urgent/elective	I	B
PVE with persisting fever and positive blood cultures >7-10 days	Urgent	I	B
PVE caused by staphylococci or gram negative bacteria (most cases of early PVE)	Urgent/elective	IIa	C
C- PREVENTION OF EMBOLISM			
PVE with recurrent emboli despite appropriate antibiotic treatment	Urgent	I	B
PVE with large vegetations (>10mm) and other predictors of complicated course (heart failure, persistent infection, abscess)	Urgent	I	C
PVE with isolated very large vegetations (>15mm)	urgent	IIb	C

Table 4. ESC guidelines for PVE

8. Right heart endocarditis

Endocarditis can affect the tricuspid valve, pulmonary valve, right ventricle or right atrium and accounts for up to 10% of cases. Predisposing risk factors for right sided endocarditis include intravenous drug abuse and the presence of foreign bodies such as pacemaker leads, haemodialysis catheters, other central venous catheters and valvular prostheses. Congenital anomalies such as ventricular septal defects and bicuspid pulmonary valves also predispose to right heart endocarditis.

Right heart endocarditis is characterised by large, friable vegetations which embolise readily to the pulmonary circulation. The resultant lung abscesses occasionally rupture causing empyema and bronchopleural fistula (see Figure 6). Staphylococcus aureus is the dominant organism, but fungal and Gram negative infections also occur.

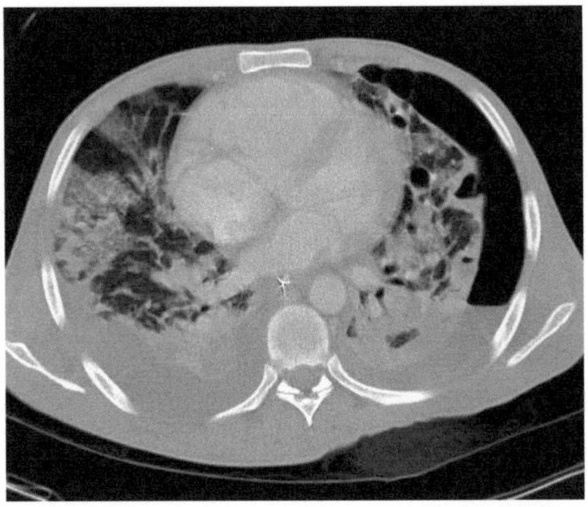

Figure 6. Computed tomography scan demonstrating florid embolic lung abscesses with cavitation, bronchopleural fistula and pyopneumothorax in a patient with pulmonary valve endocarditis due to Staphylococcus aureus.

Clinical manifestations are typically those of fever and respiratory distress, but severe haemodynamic compromise and shock may occasionally occur due to sepsis, rather than direct effects on valvular heart function. [33]

Decision making in right heart endocarditis is often problematic, because the indications for surgery are less well defined than for left-sided endocarditis. Many cases can be managed successfully without the need for surgical intervention; however large vegetations (>2cm), fungal infection, heart failure and intractable sepsis should prompt consideration for operative intervention. [33-35, 9] Table 5 summarises the indications for surgery in RSE according to the ESC guidelines.

Recommendations: right-sided endocarditis	Class	Level
Surgical treatment should be considered in the following scenarios: • Microorganisms difficult to eradicate (e.g. persistent fungi) or bacteraemia for >7 days (e.g. *S. aureus, P. aeruginosa*) despite adequate antiomicrobila therapy or • Persistent tricuspid valve vegetations >20mm after recurrent pulmonary emboli with or without concomitant right heart failure or • Right heart failure secondary to severe tricuspid regurgitation with poor response to diuretic therapy	IIa	C

Table 5. ESC guidelines for right-sided endocarditis

In cases of infected transvenous pacemaker leads, percutaneous removal is generally recommended, despite the risk of dislodging vegetations and causing pulmonary embolism. Surgery is reserved for cases where percutaneous removal is incomplete or impossible, where vegetations are very large (>25mm) or where there is associated severe destructive tricuspid valve disease. [9]

The principles of surgery for right heart endocarditis are similar to left-sided disease, namely thorough debridement of infected and necrotic tissue, removal of all infected foreign material and valvular reconstruction or replacement as required. Many cases of tricuspid valve endocarditis can be treated successfully with vegetectomy and valve repair, but replacement may be necessary with more extensive infection.

Because of the risk of recurrent infection in intravenous drug abusers, valve replacement should be avoided whenever possible in this patient group. If replacement is necessary, future compliance with anticoagulation becomes an important consideration when deciding upon mechanical versus bioprosthetic valves. An alternative is valvectomy without replacement, but the resultant free valvular regurgitation may not be tolerated acutely in some patients and late results are less satisfactory.

9. Results of surgery

The contemporary results of surgery for infective endocarditis indicate that this is still a difficult surgical condition with substantial risk of postoperative morbidity and mortality.

The Cleveland Clinic reported a series of 428 patients undergoing surgery between 2003 and 2007 with an overall hospital mortality of 10%. [32] Prosthetic valve endocarditis had a significantly higher mortality compared with NVE (13% versus 5.6%). Infection with Staphylococcus aureus also predicted a higher early and late mortality in this series.

Toronto General Hospital reported a series of 383 patients undergoing surgery for infective endocarditis over a 26-year period between 1978 and 2004. [31] Hospital mortality was 12%. Age, shock, prosthetic valve endocarditis, left ventricular ejection fraction less than 40%, and recurrent endocarditis were independent predictors of death from all causes in this series.

A multicentre prospective study of 1516 patients with NVE was published by Cabell et al in 2005 [5]. Six hundred and ten patients underwent surgery and the remaining 906 were treated medically. Hospital mortality was similar in the two groups (13.6% versus 16.4%). However, propensity analysis identified a significant survival benefit for surgery (11.2% mortality versus 38%) in the subgroup with the most number of predictors for surgery, namely male gender, congestive heart failure, aortic valve involvement, and intracardiac abscess. The authors conclude that the benefits of surgery are most realised in a targeted population.

The same investigators also examined the results of treatment for PVE. [7] Of 355 patients with PVE, 148 underwent surgery and 207 received medical treatment alone. Unadjusted hospital mortality was similar in the two groups (25% versus 23.4%). Brain embolism and Staphylococcus aureus were independent predictors of mortality.

In the 2010 prospective multicentre study of NVE by Lalani et al [10] quoted earlier, mortality in 720 patients treated surgically was 12.1%. This compared favourably with the 20.7% mortality for medical treatment.

In summary, surgery for infective endocarditis is associated with an overall hospital mortality of approximately 10-20%. The risk is roughly doubled in PVE compared with NVE.

10. Summary

Surgery for infective endocarditis has evolved enormously since its origins 75 years ago. Guidelines now exist to recommend the indications, timing, and type of surgery, yet much of the evidence is founded on observational data rather than randomized clinical trials. More than perhaps any other surgical issue, decisions rely as much on the experience and judgement of the individual surgeon as the largely observational evidence accumulated in the literature. The principles of surgery remain essentially unchanged, namely the debridement of all infected and non-viable tissue. Valve replacement is the standard of care in the majority of cases, but valve sparing techniques of repair have also gradually evolved. More extensive cardiac reconstruction with root replacement and other methods are sometimes necessary in locally advanced infection. Operative mortality and morbidity is still significant, particularly for prosthetic valve endocarditis.

Acknowledgements

The authors wish to acknowledge the assistance of Ms Charlene Nell in helping obtain permissions for reproduction of copyrighted images, and the support of the Green Lane Research and Educational Fund in helping meet the costs of preparing the chapter for publication.

Author details

Nicholas Kang[1] and Warren Smith[2]

1 Green Lane Cardiothoracic Surgical Unit, Auckland, New Zealand

2 Green Lane Hospital, Auckland, New Zealand

References

[1] Wallace A, Young G, Ostenhout S. Treatment of Acute Bacterial Endocarditis by Valve Excision and Replacement. Circulation 1965;31:450-3

[2] Alexi-Meskishvili VV, Böttcher W. The First Closure of the Persistent Ductus Arteriosus. Ann Thorac Surg 2010;90:349 –56

[3] Wilcox BR, Anderson RH. Surgical anatomy of the heart. 2nd ed. Gower Medical Publishing. London

[4] Muresian H. The Ross Procedure: New Insights Into the Surgical Anatomy Ann Thorac Surg 2006;81:495-501

[5] Cabell CH, Abrutyn E, Fowler VG Jr, Hoen B, Miro JM, Corey GR, Olaison L, Pappas P, Anstrom KJ, Stafford JA, Eykyn S, Habib G, Mestres CA, Wang A. Use of surgery in patients with native valve infective endocarditis: results from the International Collaboration on Endocarditis Merged Database. International Collaboration on Endocarditis Merged Database (ICE-MD) Study Group Investigators. Am Heart J. 2005 Nov;150(5):1092-8.

[6] Tornos P, Iung B, Permanyer-Miralda G, Baron G, Delahaye F, Gohlke-Bärwolf Ch, Butchart EG, Ravaud P, Vahanian A. Infective endocarditis in Europe: lessons from the Euro heart survey. Heart. 2005;91:571-5.

[7] Wang A, Pappas P, Anstrom KJ, Abrutyn E, Fowler VG Jr, Hoen B, Miro JM, Corey GR, Olaison L, Stafford JA, Mestres CA, Cabell CH; International Collaboration on Endocarditis Investigators. The use and effect of surgical therapy for prosthetic valve infective endocarditis: a propensity analysis of a multicenter, international cohort. Am Heart J. 2005 Nov;150(5):1086-91.

[8] Bonow RO, Carabello BA, Chatterjee K, et al. 2008 Focused update incorporated into the ACC/AHA 2006 guidelines for the management of patients with valvular heart disease: a report of the American College of Cardiology/American Heart Association Task Force on Practice Guidelines (Writing Committee to revise the 1998 guidelines for the management of patients with valvular heart disease): endorsed by the Society of Cardiovascular Anesthesiologists, Society for Cardiovascular Angiography and Interventions, and Society of Thoracic Surgeons. American College of Cardiology/ American Heart Association Task Force on Practice Guidelines. J Am Coll Cardiol 2008;52(13):e1-e142.

[9] Habib G, Hoen B, Tornos P, et al. Guidelines on the prevention, diagnosis, and treatment of infective endocarditis (new version 2009): the Task Force on the Prevention, Diagnosis, and Treatment of Infective Endocarditis of the European Society of Cardiology (ESC). Eur Heart J 2009;30:2369-413.

[10] Lalani T, Cabell CH, Benjamin DK, Lasca O, Naber C, Fowler VG Jr, Corey GR, Chu VH, Fenely M, Pachirat O, Tan RS, Watkin R, Ionac A, Moreno A, Mestres CA, Casabé J, Chipigina N, Eisen DP, Spelman D, Delahaye F, Peterson G, Olaison L, Wang A. International Collaboration on Endocarditis-Prospective Cohort Study (ICE-PCS)Investigators. Analysis of the impact of early surgery on in-hospital mortality of

native valve endocarditis: use of propensity score and instrumental variable methods to adjust for treatment-selection bias. Circulation. 2010 Mar 2;121(8):1005-13.

[11] Farzaneh-Far R, Bolger AF. Surgical Timing in Infectious Endocarditis. Wrestling With the Unrandomized. Circulation. 2010;121:960-2

[12] Vikram HR, Buenconsejo J, Hasbun R, Quagliarello VJ. Impact of valve surgery on 6-month mortality in adults with complicated, left-sided native valve endocarditis: a propensity analysis. JAMA. 2003;290:3207–3214.

[13] Kang DH, Kim YJ, Kim SH, Sun BJ, Kim DH, Yun SC, Song JM, Choo SJ, Chung CH, Song JK, Lee JW, Sohn DW. Early surgery versus conventional treatment for infective endocarditis. N Engl J Med. 2012 Jun 28;366(26):2466-73.

[14] Thuny F, Disalvo G, Belliard O, Avierinos JF, Pergola V, Rosenberg V, Casalta JP, Gouvernet J, Derumeaux G, Iarussi D, Ambrosi P, Calabro R, Riberi A, Collart F, Metras D, Lepidi H, Raoult D, Harle JR, Weiller PJ, Cohen A, Habib G. Risk of embolism and death in infective endocarditis: prognostic value of echocardiography: a prospective multicenter study. Circulation. 2005;112:69 –75.

[15] Vilacosta I, Graupner C, San Román JA, Sarriá C, Ronderos R, Fernández C, Mancini L, Sanz O, Sanmartín JV, Stoermann W. Risk of embolization after institution of antibiotic therapy for infective endocarditis. J Am Coll Cardiol. 2002;39:1489-95.

[16] Fabri J Jr, Issa VS, Pomerantzeff PM, Grinberg M, Barretto AC, Mansur AJ. Time-related distribution, risk factors and prognostic influence of embolism in patients with left-sided infective endocarditis. Int J Cardiol. 2006;110:334-9.

[17] Rossi M, Gallo A, De Silva RJ, Sayeed R. What is the optimal timing for surgery in infective endocarditis with cerebrovascular complications? Interact Cardiovasc Thorac Surg. 2012;14:72-80.

[18] Lee LS, Chen FY, Cohn LH. Management of native valve endocarditis. In Sabiston and Spencer Surgery of the Chest 8th ed Sellke, del Nido, Swanson

[19] Pavie A. Heart transplantation for end-stage valvular disease: indications and results Curr Opin Cardiol 2006;21:100–105

[20] Feringa HH, Shaw LJ, Poldermans D, Hoeks S, van der Wall EE, Dion RA, Bax JJ. Mitral valve repair and replacement in endocarditis: a systematic review of literature. Ann Thorac Surg. 2007;83:564-70.

[21] Evans CF, Gammie JS. Surgical management of mitral valve infective endocarditis. Semin Thorac Cardiovasc Surg. 2011;23:232-40

[22] Mayer K, Aicher D, Feldner S, Kunihara T, Schäfers HJ. Repair versus replacement of the aortic valve in active infective endocarditis. Eur J Cardiothorac Surg. 2012;42:122-7

[23] Haydock D, Barratt-Boyes B, Macedo T, Kirklin JW, Blackstone E. Aortic valve replacement for active infectious endocarditis in 108 patients. A comparison of free-

hand allograft valves with mechanical prostheses and bioprostheses. J Thorac Cardiovasc Surg. 1992;103(1):130-9.

[24] Sabik JF, Lytle BW, Blackstone EH, Marullo AG, Pettersson GB, Cosgrove DM. Aortic root replacement with cryopreserved allograft for prosthetic valve endocarditis. Ann Thorac Surg. 2002;74:650-9

[25] Edwards MB, Ratnatunga CP, Dore CJ, Taylor KM. Thirty-day mortality and long-term survival following surgery for prosthetic endocarditis: a study from the UK heart valve registry. Eur J Cardiothorac Surg 1998;14:156–164.

[26] Bozbuga N, Erentug V, Erdogan HB, Kirali K, Ardal H, Tas S, Akinci E, Yakut C. Tex Heart Inst J. 2004;31(4):382-6. Surgical treatment of aortic abscess and fistula.

[27] Avierinos J-F, Thuny F, Chalvignac V, et al. Surgical treatment of active aortic endocarditis: homografts are not the cornerstone of outcome. Ann Thorac Surg 2007;84:1935-42.

[28] Hagl C, Galla JD, Lansman SL. Replacing the ascending aorta and aortic valve for acute prosthetic valve endocarditis: is using prosthetic material contraindicated? Ann Thorac Surg 2002;74:S1781-5.

[29] David TE, Feindel CM. Reconstruction of the mitral annulus. Circulation 1987;76:III102-107.

[30] Prendergast BD, Tornos P. Surgery for infective endocarditis: who and when? Circulation. 2010;121:1141-52.

[31] David TE, Gavra G, Feindel CM, Regesta T, Armstrong S, Maganti MD. Surgical treatment of active infective endocarditis: a continued challenge. J Thorac Cardiovasc Surg 2007;133:144–149.

[32] Manne MB, Shrestha NK, Lytle BW, et al. Outcomes after surgical treatment of native and prosthetic valve infective endocarditis. Ann Thorac Surg 2012;93:489-93.

[33] Kang N, Smith W, Greaves S, Haydock D. Pulmonary valve endocarditis. N Engl J Med. 2007;356:2224-5.

[34] Robbins MJ, Frater RW, Soeiro R, Frishman WH, Strom JA. Influence of vegetation size on clinical outcome of right-sided infective endocarditis. Am J Med 1986;80:165-71.

[35] Hecht SR, Berger M. Right-sided endocarditis in intravenous drug users: prognostic features in 102 episodes. Ann Intern Med 1992;117:560-6

Chapter 6

New Treatment Modalities for Ocular Complications of Endocarditis

Ozlem Sahin

Additional information is available at the end of the chapter

http://dx.doi.org/10.5772/56537

1. Introduction

Endophthalmitis is one of the most devastating diagnoses in ophthalmology. It is a serious intraocular inflammatory disorder affecting the vitreous cavity that can result from exogenous or endogenous spread of infecting organisms into the eye. [1] Endogenous endophthalmitis is less common and occurs secondary to hematogenous dissemination from a distant infective source in the body. Predisposing risk factors in patients with endogenous endophthalmitis usually exist, and they are correlated with the pathogenesis of the disease.[1] The risk factors are considered as infectious foci in the other parts of the body, intravenous drug abuse, diabetes mellitus, immunosuppressive therapy, intravenous hyperalimentation, fever of unknown origin, malignancies and male sex. [2-6] In most cases, independent of its origin, the presentation of endophthalmitis consists of reduced or blurred vision, red eye, pain, and lid swelling. [7] Progressive vitritis (Fig.1) is one of the key findings in any form of endophthalmitis, and in nearly 75% of patients have hypopyon (Fig. 2) which can be seen at the time of presentation. [7] Progression of the disease may lead to panophthalmitis, (Fig. 3) corneal infiltration, (Fig. 4) globe perforation and phthisis bulbi.(Fig. 5) [1,7] Endogenous endophthalmitis is a rare complication of infective endocarditis, and has been decreasing due to the availability of effective antibiotics. [8] To optimize visual outcome, early diagnosis and treatment are essential.[7,8] Over recent decades, advances in hygienic standards, improved microbiologic and surgical techniques, development of powerful antimicrobial drugs, and the introduction of intravitreal antibiotic therapy have led to a decreased incidence and improved management of endophthalmitis. [1,7] However, endophthalmitis still represents a serious clinical problem. This chapter focuses mainly on current principles and techniques for treatment of endophthalmitis. In addition, it addresses recent developments regarding anti-inflammatory and antimicrobial treatments.

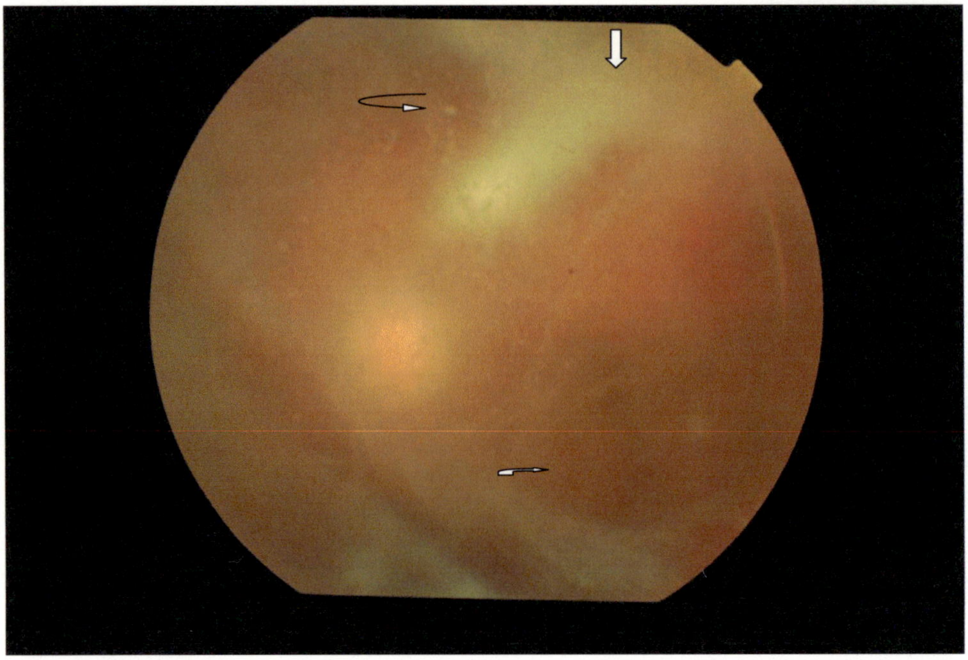

Figure 1. Note the dense vitritis, vitreous bands, ( ) precipitates, ( ) and retinitis foci ( ) located superiorly.

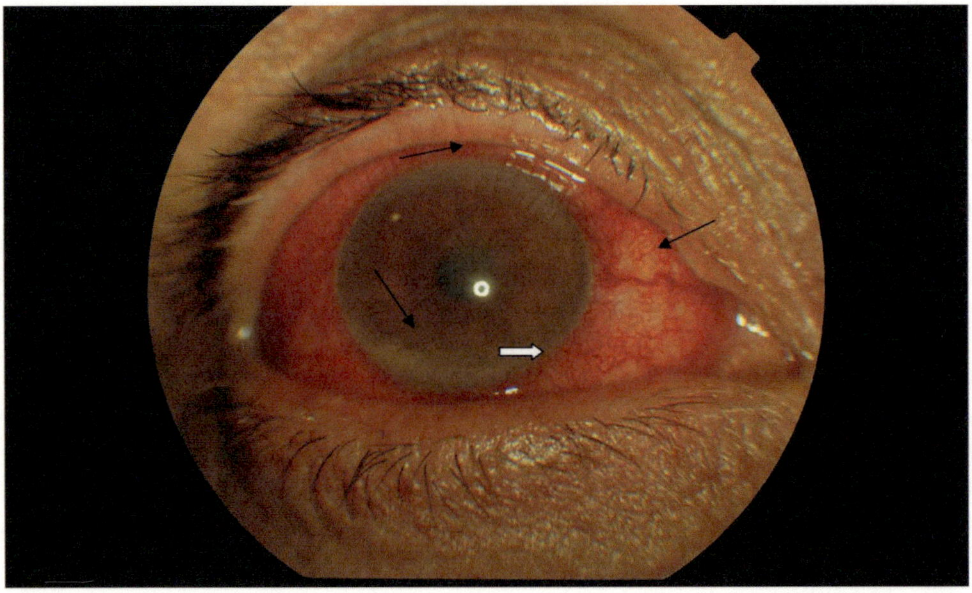

Figure 2. Note the 2-mm hypopyon ( ) in the anterior chamber associated with diffuse ciliary injection ( )

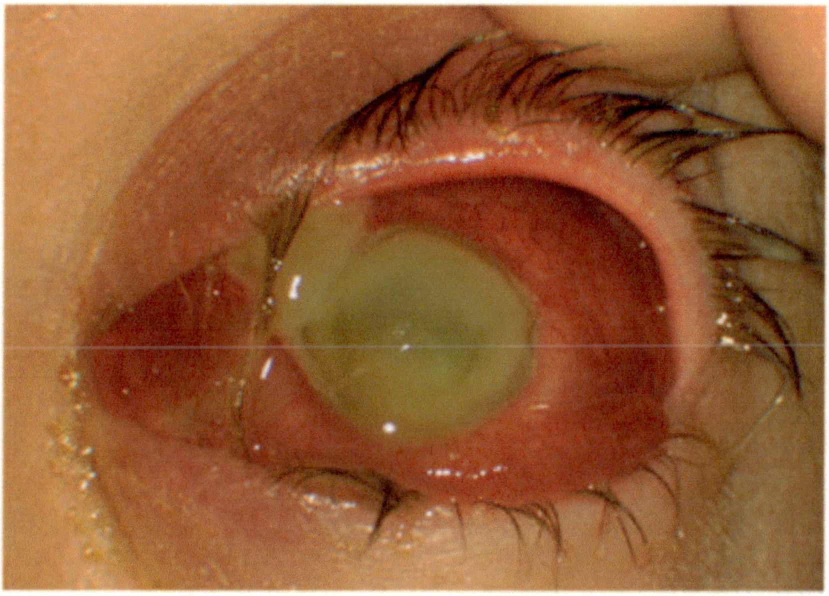

Figure 3. Note severe panophthalmitis with superonasal scleral abscess, and extrusion of pus from the limbus. (A Shwe-Tin, T Ung, C Madhavan and T Yasen: A case of endogenous Clostridium perfringens endophthalmitis in an intravenous drug abuser. Eye (2007) 21, 1427–1428; doi:10.1038/sj.eye.6702934; published online 3 August 2007)

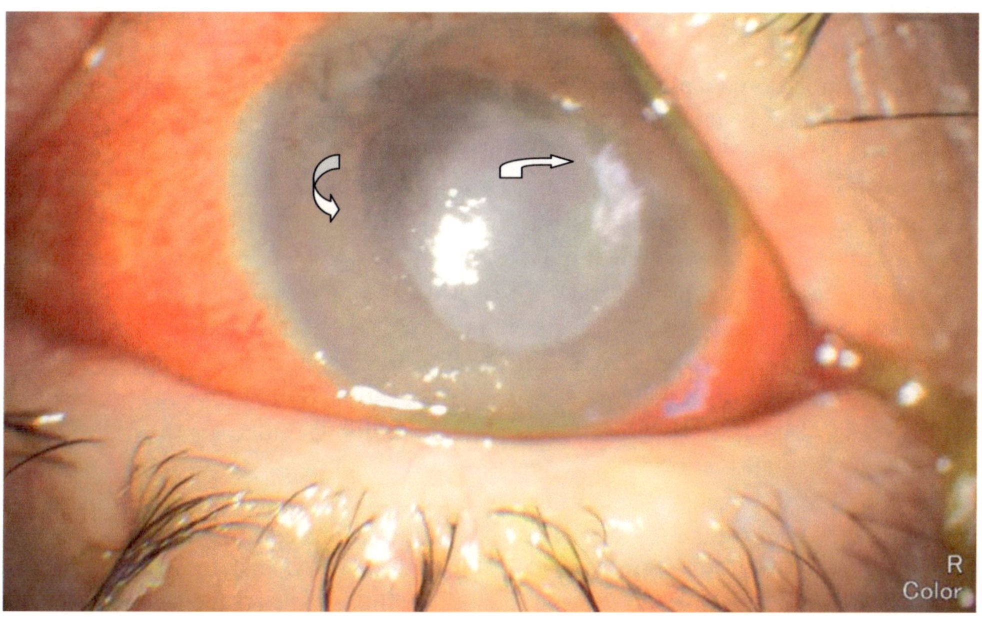

Figure 4. Note the central corneal infiltration ( ) and diffuse stromal edema ( )

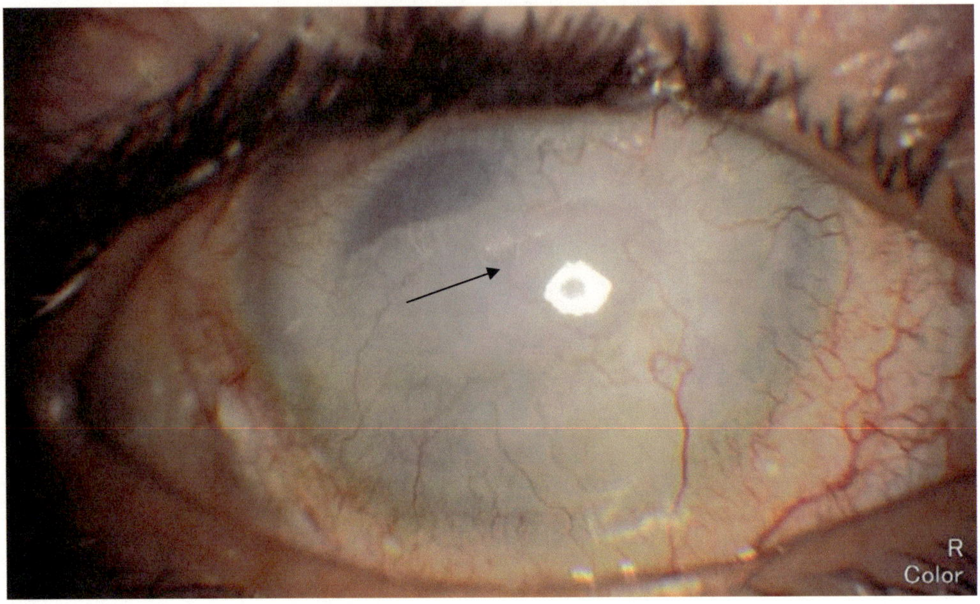

Figure 5. Note the phytisis bulbi associated with diffuse corneal vascularization and opacification (⟶)

2. Pathogenesis

In general, inflammation is a physiological response to invading pathogens or antigens which involve the migration of specific types of inflammatory cells out of the bloodstream into theaffected tissues. [9,10] These cells release inflammatory agents such as cytokines, chemokines and other inflammatory markers to boost immune responses to kill the invading bacteria, viruses, and parasites or any other antigen. [9,10] The linking of the antibody to the antigens forms an immune complex which is removed quickly by phagocytic macrophages; however owing to excessive antigen exposure or compromised immune response, the pathogens or their toxins are lodged into tissues and cause severe inflammation. [11,12] Excessive inflammatory response can damage the healthy tissues during this process. In excessive inflammation, the affected parts of the eye (the eyelids, sclera, iris, uvea, retina, optic nerve etc) become tender and inflamed. [11,12] Chronic or sever ocular inflammation can damage the delicate tissues and blood vessels in and around the eye resulting in vision loss. [13] Ocular inflammatory diseases occurs throughout the world independent of gender, race, ethnicity, or age and can be caused due to various factors such as infection, auto-immunity, trauma, drugs, or malignancy. [13] As the infectious pathogens enter the eye via hematogenous spread bacterial endotoxins, cytokins and growth factors induce the cellular mechanisms of reactive oxygen species (ROS) formation. [14] The key mediators are hydrogen peroxide (H_2O_2), superoxide anions and peroxinitrite (NOO–), collectively termed as ROS. [14-16] ROS are believed to underlie many of the oxidative changes in various pathological conditions, and are known to enhance various mediators including increased expression of aldose reductase (AR), activation of protein kinase C and redox-sensitive nuclear transcription factors such as NF-κB and activator protein-1 (AP-1). [15-17] ROS in turn lead to the cell membrane lipid peroxidation and formation of lipid aldehydes, e.g. 4-hydroxynonenal-(HNE) which conjugates with glutathione. (GS-HNE) Aldose reductase then catalyzes reduction of GS-HNE into glutathione 1,4 dihydroxynonene (GS-DHN) which acts as a transducer of inflammatory signaling by activating protein kinases system.[18,19] Eventually, the redox-sensitive transcription factors including NF-κB and AP-1 are activated in the nucleus, and transcribe many inflammatory genes that contribute to intraocular inflammation such as endophthalmitis. [19-21] Many inflammatory mediators, such as TNF-α, IL-1β, IL-6, and inducible-nitric oxide synthase (iNOS) require NF-κB activation for their expression as their genes possess NF-κB binding sequences in promoter regions. [19-21] Since the discovery of NF-κB, a number of paradigms for its function have been established including its key role in the inflammatory and immune responses. NF-κB stimulates immune cell function and acts in a pro-inflammatory manner by inducing the expression of cytokines, chemokines and their receptors. [19-21]These aspects of NF-κB function are undoubtedly central to the understanding of the overall action of this family of transcription factors, and they provide a foundation for therapeutic intervention in inflammatory diseases based on NF-κB inhibition. [22,23] AR mediates the activation of NF-κB during oxidative stress caused by various stimuli and that inhibition of AR attenuates the activation of key signaling kinases leading to deactivation of NF-κB. It is plausible that AR inhibitors could be potential therapeutic agents to treat the oxidative stress-induced ocular inflammation. [22,23] Alternatively, it has been shown that inhibition of AR prevents NF-κB activation in both cellular as well as animal models of ocular inflammation, thereby regulating the synthesis and secretion of pro-inflammatory markers suggesting that inhibition of AR by gene silencing or pharmacological agents could be an important strategy to treat ocular inflammatory diseases. [24,25] The evidence showing that lipid peroxidation products are being the excellent substrates of AR has led to this enzyme linked to inflammation and auto-immune mediated oxidative stress, besides diabetic complications. [26,27] Many studies with cell-culture and animal models of ocular inflammation have shown that inhibition of AR could ameliorate the inflammation induced by various stimuli including bacterial endotoxin, lipopolysachharide (LPS), high glucose, and cytokines. [24-27]The increased expression of AR in human cornea, lens, retina, and optic nerve has been shown during oxidative stress. [28,29] More recent reports suggest an unanticipated link between AR and ocular inflammation, e.g. inhibition of AR by pharmacological agents or by mRNA ablation leads to the prevention of high glucose-, TNF-α-, and LPS-induced oxidative stress in human lens epithelial cells (HLEC) suggesting that AR could be another molecular target for the treatment of oxidative stress-induced ocular inflammation. [27] Although the eye is an immunologically privileged organ, it can also get damaged from the excessive immune response of the body when blood ocular barrier function is compromised. [30] Both in-vitro and *in-vivo* studies have demonstrated that AR inhibition or ablation prevents the activation of PKC/NF-κB thereby attenuate cytotoxicity and tissue damage. [31] It has also been shown that AR inhibition in rodent endotoxin-induced uveitis model leads to attenuation of ocular inflammation as characterized by decreased protein extravasations and cellular infiltration into the anterior chamber [24]. These results demonstrated that AR inhibition leads to in-vivo suppression of NF-κB that can attenuate inflammation in the eye. In HLEC, it has recently been shown that AR mediates the LPS-induced cytotoxicity via the activation of redox sensitive transcription factors NF-κB and AP-1, and inhibition of AR by pharmacological inhibitor or by silencing the AR expression by AR siRNA prevented the cytotoxicity caused by LPS. [32] These findings are significant as LPS – induced ocular inflammation, such as endogenous endophthalmitis in which infection reaches the eye via circulation and infection-induced uveitis, are well known threats to vision in humans. [33,34] Inhibition of such inflammation by AR inhibitors provides a novel therapeutic approach for infection –induced ocular diseases. Further, a study by Kubo et al showed that over-expression AR in HLEC led to the increased oxidative stress and apoptosis, and inhibition of AR prevented the cells from oxidative stres. [35] In a recent study, it has been demonstrated that AR mediates LPS-induced cytotoxicity in non-pigmented ciliary epithelial cells and disturbs the aqueous humor dynamics by altering the expression of channel proteins such as Na-K-ATPase. [36] This study has greater implication in the infection-induced ocular inflammation as reduced flow of aqueous humor could result in severe vision impairment or vision loss. Besides, attraction of macrophages to the ocular tissues or activation of resident macrophages e.g. dendritic cells during inflammation cause severe damage to the ciliary body and retinal layers. [33-35] The role of AR in LPS-induced inflammation and macrophage activation is important because macrophages play an important role in the ocular inflammation such as uveitis. Macrophages infiltrate the vasculature and enter the aqueous humor in anterior segment releasing enormous amount of cytokines and chemokines that result in the pathological symptoms of uveitis such as flare, cell, edema, and vasodilation. [37] Therefore, it is significant in the way that AR inhibition provides a novel therapeutic target in ocular inflammatory diseases. Studies in the cellular models provide an evidence of an unanticipated role of AR in mediating acute inflammatory responses, and also inhibition of AR might be therapeutically useful in preventing ocular inflammation induced by oxidative stress especially in various pathological conditions.

3. Basic principles in the treatment of endogenous

3.1. Endophthalmitis

The therapy of infectious endophthalmitis remains a controversial issue because progression and suboptimal outcome occur despite bacteriologic cure of the intraocular infection. The irreversible tissue destruction during the inflammatory process may result largely from a secondary host inflammatory response. However, adjunctive treatment with immunosuppressive agents may interfere with the ability of the immune system to eliminate the microorganisms. Hence the option of adjunctive immunosuppression in the therapy of infectious endophthalmitis is still on debate. Endogenous endophthalmitis is treated by a combination of broad-spectrum antibiotics (vancomycin and ceftazidime or amikacin), which are administered intravitreally, subconjunctivally and topically, if appropriate in combination by systemic antibiotics (vancomycin and ceftazidime or amikacin). [1,2] If vision diminishes to mere light perception, performance of pars plana vitrectomy is indicated. [2-4] In mycotic endophthalmitis, antimycotics (amphotericin B) are administered intravitreally. [38,39] If findings are severe, a pars plana vitrectomy must also be carried out. [40,41] Antimycotics are applied topically to support treatment. [38] Systemic therapy with antibiotics or mycotics is obligatory. [42]

3.2. Topical antimicrobial agents

Fluoroquinolones are especially useful because they possess a broad antibacterial spectrum, bactericidal in action, are generally well tolerated, and have been less prone to development of bacterial resistance. [43]

Second-generation fluoroquinolones; Ciprofloxacin 0.3% and Ofloxacin 0.3% have been widely used in the treatment and prophylaxis of ocular infections. [43,44] However, their in-vitro potencies have been decreasing steadily since their introduction. But ciprofloxacin remains the most effective fluoroquinolone against gram-negative bacteria. Minimal inhibitory concentration at 90% level (MIC90) for ciprofloxacin is lower in gram-negative bacteria. MIC90 for ofloxacin is higher against Haemophilus spp. and Moraxella spp. Ciprofloxacin is clinically the most potent fluoroquinolone for Pseudomonas spp. Ciprofloxacin is just as potent as gatifloxacin for the other gram-negative isolates.[44]Third-generation fluoroquinolones; Levofloxacin 0.5% produces higher ocular tissue penetration, thereby reducing the risk of selecting for decreased fluoroquinolone potency. A new third-generation formulation, levofloxacin 1.5%, is recently introduced, demonstrating increased ocular penetration compared with gatifloxacin 0.3%, but clinical equivalence to its second-generation parent, ofloxacin 0.3%, in two randomized trials. [45]Fourth-generation fluoroquinolones; Fourth-generation agents have increased potency against gram-positive bacteria compared with levofloxacin, while maintaining similar potency against gram-negative bacteria. [46] Although levofloxacin 1.5% has demonstrated superior ocular penetration relative to gatifloxacin, the limited available data do not suggest this translates into superior clinical activity compared with moxifloxacin, which has significantly greater ocular penetration and better gram-positive potency than gatifloxacin. [46] Gatifloxacin 0.3% and moxifloxacin 0.5% have structural modifications that both reduce risk of resistance and improve potency against gram-positive bacteria. Fourth-generation agents have increased potency against gram-positive bacteria compared with levofloxacin, while maintaining similar potency against gram-negative bacteria. [47] From susceptibility profiles achieved with in vitro testing, the fourth-generation fluoroquinolones may offer some advantages over the currently available fluoroquinolones; however, a combination of the pharmacodynamics and pharmacokinetics of the drug, infection site, and the MIC90 is needed to predict the in vivo efficacy and best clinical applicability. [47] The fourth-generation fluoroquinolones are clinically more potent than the second generations for gram-positive bacteria. The MIC90 level is lower for moxifloxacin than that for gatifloxacin against Staphylococcus aureus, methicillin-susceptible coagulase-negative Staphylococcus (CoNS), and Streptococcus pneumoniae, whereas the levels are equal against Streptococcus viridans and the gatifloxacin MIC90 is lower in methicillin-resistant coagulase-negative CoNS [48] With in vitro tests, Staphylococcus aureus isolates that are resistant to ciprofloxacin and ofloxacin are clinicallymost susceptible to moxifloxacin. CoNS, that are resistant to ciprofloxacin and ofloxacin are clinically most susceptible to moxifloxacin and gatifloxacin. [48]Streptococcus viridans are more susceptible to moxifloxacin, gatifloxacin and levofloxacin than ciprofloxacin and ofloxacin. Streptococcus pneumoniae is least susceptible to ofloxacin compared with the other fluoroquinolones. [48] Susceptibilities are found equivalent for all other bacterial groups. In general, moxifloxacin is the most potent fluoroquinolone for gram-positive bacteria, while ciprofloxacin, moxifloxacin, gatifloxacin, and levofloxacin demonstrate equivalent potencies to gram-negative bacteria. [45,47] None of the fluoroquinolones are effective against ciprofloxacin-resistant gram-negative bacteria. Overall, for gram-positive bacteria, median MIC90s of levofloxacin, moxifloxacin and gatifloxacin are below ciprofloxacin, the MIC90 of gatifloxacin and moxifloxacin is equal for gram-positive bacteria. Levofloxacin, gatifloxacin and moxifloxacin are clinically more effective against gram-positive bacteria, the latter two being equally effective. Ciprofloxacin remains the most effective fluoroquinolone against gram-negative bacteria. [45,48] Fourth-generation fluoroquinolone moxifloxacin, seems to have better penetration to the inflamed ocular tissues in rabbit. [49] Moxifloxacin has a spectrum of coverage that encompasses the most common organisms in endophthalmitis. [49] Because of their broad spectrum of coverage, low MIC90, good tolerability, and excellent oral bioavailability, fourth-generation fluoroquinolones are considered to represent a major advance for managing posterior segment infections. [47,49]

Delivery of moxifloxacin via a collagen shield is recommended when high concentrations of moxifloxacin are most needed to clear the aqueous of bacteria. [50] There are several advantages of this route of delivery that make it appealing over the frequent topical drop use in the immediate period. [50] Future studies are considered to define precisely the role of fourth-generation fluoroquinolones and presoaked collagen shields in the prophylaxis or management of intraocular infections.

Orally administered gatifloxacin achieves therapeutic levels in the noninflamed human eye, and the activity spectrum appropriately encompass the bacterial species most frequently involved in the various causes of endophthalmitis. Because of its broad-spectrum coverage, low MIC90 levels for the organisms of concern, and good tolerability, gatifloxacin represents a major advance in the prophylaxis or treatment of bacterial endophthalmitis including Staphylococcus epidermidis, Staphylococcus aureus, Streptococcus pneumoniae, Streptococcus pyogenes, Propionibacterium acnes, Haemophilus influenzae, Escherichia coli, Bacillus cereus, Proteus mirabilis, and other organisms. [51] Besifloxacin, the latest advanced fluoroquinolone approved for treating bacterial conjunctivitis is the first fluoroquinolone developed specifically for topical ophthalmic use. [52] It has a C-8 chlorine substituent and is known as a chloro-fluoroquinolone. Besifloxacin possesses relatively balanced dual-targeting activity against bacterial topoisomerase IV and DNA gyrase (topoisomerse II), two essential enzymes involved in bacterial DNA replication, leading to increased potency and decreased likelihood of bacterial resistance developing to besifloxacin. [52] Microbiological data suggest a relatively high potency and rapid bactericidal activity for besifloxacin against common ocular pathogens, including bacteria resistant to other fluoroquinolones, especially resistant staphylococcal species. [52,53] Randomized, double-masked, controlled clinical studies demonstrated the clinical efficacy of besifloxacin ophthalmic suspension 0.6% administered three-times daily for

5 days to be superior to the vehicle alone and similar to moxifloxacin ophthalmic solution 0.5% for bacterial conjunctivitis. [53] In addition, besifloxacin ophthalmic suspension 0.6% administered two-times daily for 3 days isclinically more effective than the vehicle alone for bacterial conjunctivitis. Besifloxacin has also been shown in preclinical animal studies to be potentially effective for the "off-label" treatment of infections following ocular surgery, prophylaxis of endophthalmitis, and the treatment of bacterial keratitis. Taken together, clinical and preclinical animal studies indicate that besifloxacin is an important new option for the treatment of ocular infections. [53]Both besifloxacin and moxifloxacin achieved aqueous humor concentrations equal to or slightly higher than their respective MIC90 for methicillin-resistant and methicillin-susceptible Staphylococcus aureus and Staphylococcus epidermidis; none of the fluoroquinolones achieved concentrations above their MIC90 for ciprofloxacin-resistant strains of Staphylococcus aureus and Staphylococcus epidermidis. [54] Based on the aqueous humor drug concentrations measured, it is unlikely that any of the fluoroquinolones tested would be therapeutically effective in the aqueous humor against the most frequently identified drug-resistant Staphylococcal isolates from cases of endophthalmitis. [54] As well as; none of the fluoroquinolones reduce the number of bacteria recovered from the vitreous humor. [54] Besifloxacin is as effective as moxifloxacin and gatifloxacin in a rabbit model for topical prophylaxis and treatment of pneumococcal endophthalmitis. [55] Besifloxacin acts as an anti-inflammatory agent in corneal epithelial cells in vitro, by inhibiting the nuclear factor, NF-κB and mitogen-activated protein kinase (MAPK) pathways. Besifloxacin also exhibits anti-inflammatory efficacy in vivo. [56]The anti-inflammatory attribute may enhance its efficacy in the treatment of ocular infections with an inflammatory component and warrants further investigation. [56] The newer topical fluoroquinolones gemifloxacin and pazufloxacin are considered as effective as moxifloxacin and levofloxacin for topical prophylaxis and for the treatment of Staphylococcus aureus-induced endophthalmitis in the rabbit model. [57]

Early diagnosis and appropriate treatment with intravitreous antibiotics are the most important factors for the successful management of endophthalmitis. [58,59] The intraocular concentration of antibiotics after intravitreous injection is far greater than that achieved by topical modalities. Drug combinations are necessary to cover the full range of bacteria causing endophthalmitis. [58,59] Vancomycin (1 mg/0.1 ml) is considered the drug of choice for gram-positive organisms. Controversy remains concerning the best choice against gram-negative bacteria. Aminoglycosides (amikacin, 0.4 mg/0.1 ml) have traditionally been recommended for gram-negative coverage. However, because of their possible role in macular toxicity, recent trends have shifted to using ceftazidime (2.25 mg/0.1 ml) in combination with vancomycin. [59] Intracameral or intravitreal cefuroxime at a dose of 1 mg is considered effective in the treatment of endophthalmitis. [60] Electroretinographic (ERG) and histologic findings indicated that a dose of 1 mg cefuroxime, administered intravitreally, is not toxic to the rabbit retina. [60] A dose of 10 mg, injected intravitreally, induce transient physiological effects, and is toxic to the rabbit retina, as was evident by the permanent reduction in the ERG responses and by the structural damage to the retina with signs of glial activation. [60] The long-term outcomes of early intravitreal treatment of endogenous bacterial endophthalmitis, defined as intravitreal and systemic antibiotics administered within 24 h of diagnosis, with conservative use of pars plana vitrectomy is considered to provide a relatively favourable visual prognosis.

[61] The longer the time between onset of ocular symptoms and intravitreal antibiotic injection is correlated with worse visual outcomes, and it is also associated with increased mortality. [61] Mortality is also associated with methicillin-resistant Staphylococcus aureus infection. [61] Methicillin-resistant Sthapylococcus aureus isolates are reported sensitive to vancomycin, and 68% were sensitive to the fourth-generation fluoroquinolones. [62] No significant differences are reported in visual acuity outcomes of endophthalmitis caused by methicillin-sensitive Sthaphylococcus aureus versus methicillin-resistant Staphylococcus aureus treated early intravitreal vancomycin and either ceftazidime or amikacin.[62] Adjunt use of intravitreal dexamethasone in endogenous endophthalmitis is recommended. [63] No adverse events is attributed to the dexamethasone, and it appears safe and may be of benefit in endogenous endophthalmitis. [63] The advantage of corticotherapy combined with specific anti-infective treatment has been proven for certain bacterial and fungal infections. Corticosteroids, even in short-term treatments, is recommended to be prescribed in combination with antibiotics in the course of infections related to their ability to limit the deleterious effects caused by the activation of the immune system at the time of certain infections.[64] Such as; Bacillus cereus causes the most virulent and refractory form of endophthalmitis. Eyes treated with intravitreal vancomycin in conjunction with dexamethasone injection at 7 days and 14 days show significantly less inflammation over iris and vitreous than the eyes treated with intravitreal vancomycin injection alone.[65] Additionally, at 14 days, the histopathological changes of eyes treated with vancomycin with dexamethasone show less conjunctival inflammation, mild iridocyclitis, less vitreous cells, and less choroidal vasculitis and retinitis compared to the vancomycin treatment alone. [65] Intravitreal injection of vancomycin is considered to improve the therapeutic outcome of Bacillus cereus endophthalmitis. However, the addition of dexamethasone to antibiotic treatment is reported to provide a therapeutic benefit over antibiotic alone. [65]

The fluocinolone acetonide intravitreal implants a sustained drug delivery implant has been used for patients with posterior uveitis who do not respond to or are intolerant to conventional treatment. [66] It effectively controls the intraocular inflammation. Visual acuity generally improves, uveitis recurrences, and the need for immunosuppression decreases. However, the most common side effect is increased intraocular pressure, and cataract development is also reported. [66,67] The newly approved dexamethasone implant, Ozurdex, is currently considered in the treatment of noninfectious intermediate and posterior uveitis given its efficacy, safety, and ease of use in the outpatient setting. [68]

Triamcinolone acetonide (TA) is an effective steroid drug for various retinal and choroidal diseases when delivered intravitreally. [69] It may imply an off-label use and it may be associated with ocular adverse events. Intravitreal TA is not associated with significant systemic safety risks. [69] Difluprednate 0.05% ophthalmic emulsion is a potent new topical corticosteroid that exhibits enhanced penetration, better bioavailability, rapid local metabolism and strong efficacy, with a low incidence of adverse effects. In June 2008, difluprednate ophthalmic emulsion 0.05% gained FDA approval in the U.S. for the treatment of postoperative ocular inflammation and pain. Recently, a multicenter, randomized clinical trial showed difluprednate to be noninferior to prednisolone acetate 1% dosed twice as often, the current standard of care for the acute management of endogenous uveitis in the U.S. Furthermore, difluprednate proved to have a comparable safety profile. [70]

Intravitreous amphotericin B injection associated with, pars plana vitrectomy, systemic amphotericin B therapy, and oral anti-fungal therapy are indicated in the treatment of endogenous fungal endophthalmitis. [71,72] The most common cause of culture-proven endogenous fungal endophthalmitis is Candida species. [71] Endogenous Aspergillus endophthalmitis usually has an acute onset of intraocular inflammation and often has a characteristic chorioretinal lesion located in the macula. (Fig 6] [72] Although treatment with pars plana vitrectomy and intravitreous amphotericin B is capable of eliminating the ocular infection, the visual outcome generally is poor, especially when there is direct macular involvement. [72] The overall visual outcomes are reported more favorable for Candida cases than they are for Aspergillus cases. [71] Infection site, illness severity, neutropenia, hemodynamic status, organ failure and concomitant drug treatments are host-related factors that influence the choice of systemic antifungal treatment. [73] In general, echinocandins are currently favored for empiric treatment of candidemia, especially in critically ill patients or those with previous azole exposure. Essentially, patients who have been previously exposed to azoles have a higher probability of being infected by azole-resistant or non-albicans strains. [73] Pharmacokinetic properties and side effects suggest that polyenes should be avoided in patients with renal failure, and that echinocandins and azoles should be avoided in patients with severe hepatic dysfunction. [73] Intravitreal corticosteroid therapy which is also indicated in conjunction with anti-fungals with and without vitrectomy, reduces the intraocular inflammatory process and secondary complications associated with fungalendophthalmitis. [74]

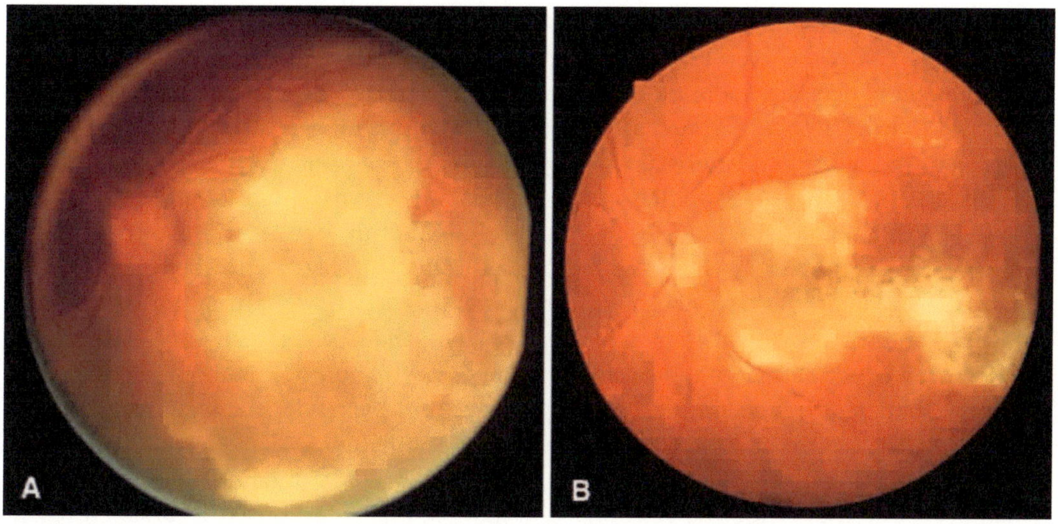

Figure 6. A. Aspergillus chorioretinal infiltrate in macula of patient with a history of intravenous drug abuse. B. After treatment with vitrectomy, intravitreal amphotericin B injection, and systemic amphotericin B, the infection resolved and a macular scar remains. (Weishaar PD, Flynn HW Jr, Murray TG et al: Endogenous Aspergillus endophthalmitis: Clinical features and treatment outcomes. Ophthalmology 105:57, 1998.)

Tumor Necrosis Factor-Alpha (TNFα) is a potent mediator of acute inflammatory reactions via activation of proinflammatory signaling cascades. [75] TNFα is a cytokine secreted by macrophages and neutrophils, and is important in upregulating cell adhesion expression on vascular endothelial cells. [75] TNFα also stimulates mononuclear phagocytes to produce cytokines, such as interlekin (IL)-1, IL-6 and itself. [75] In an experimental rat model of *Staphylococcus aureus* endophthalmitis, TNFα and IL-1β were detected in the vitreous within 6 h of intravitreal inoculation. [76] It has been shown that the upregulation of proinflammatory cytokines may have contributed to the breakdown of the blood-retina barrier, and the recruitment of neutrophils into the eye. [76] Upregulation of TNFα, IL-1β, and interferon gamma (IFNγ) have also been shown in experimental *Staphylococcus epidermidis* endophthalmitis.[77] Injection of TNFα into the vitreous of rabbits and rats induced increased vascular permeability and cellular infiltration. [78,79] Studies have also demonstrated upregulation of TNFα and other proinflammatory cytokines in experimental autoimmune uveoretinitis. [80] No studies have quantified cytokines or chemokines in the human eye during endophthalmitis, but based on experimental studies, it is reasonable to hypothesize that proinflammatory cytokines are key mediators of acute inflammation during endophthalmitis. The primary function of innate immunity is to detect invading pathogens and clear them as quickly as possible. [80] During an acute intraocular infection, a primary and essential component of this response is neutrophil influx. Cellular infiltration in human endophthalmitis cases has been described as vitritis, the presence of a hypopyon, and corneal ring abscess formation. Experimental models have identified polymorphonuclear leukocytes (PMN) as the primary infiltrating cell type during bacterial endophthalmitis.[81-84]The recruitment and activation of neutrophils within an infected eye is a biological dilemma. PMN infiltration is necessary for bacterial clearance, but the generation of toxic reactive oxygen intermediates and other inflammatory mediators by PMN may result in bystander damage to delicate tissues of the retina.[81,82] Robust inflammation is a hallmark of endophthalmitis caused by *B. cereus* and other types of virulent bacteria. In experimental *B. cereus* endophthalmitis, inflammatory cells were observed in the posterior chamber in close proximity to the optic nerve head as early as 4 h postinfection. [82] Further analysis confirms that the primary infiltrating cells are the PMNs. The numbers of $CD18^{+}/Gr\text{-}1^{+}$ PMN were minimal at 4 and 6 h postinfection, but increased significantly thereafter. The influx of $CD18^{+}/Gr\text{-}1^{+}$ PMN into the posterior segment occurred simultaneously with the increase of TNFα in the eye at approximately 4–6 h postinfection.[82] Despite their potential importance, the roles of TNFα and several other cytokines in endophthalmitis remain unexplored. Regulation of inflammation is the key to removing the pathogen without harming the eye, but bystander damage from infiltrating cells might occur. For *Staphylococcus aureus* endophthalmitis, depletion of neutrophils early in the inflammatory response reduces the severity of host inflammation, but severely hamperes bacterial clearance, resulting in a more severe infection. [81] Pathogen recognition and a well-regulated inflammatory response to infection are essential in clearing invading organisms with minimal damage to surrounding tissue. A tightly controlled response is even more critical in the eye, where non-regenerative cells and tissues responsible for vision reside. Experimental models of bacterial endophthalmitis have demonstrated that once a pathogen is introduced into the posterior segment, an acute response occurs, including synthesis of proinflammatory cytokines and influx of PMN into the eye.[83,84] In the case of virulent pathogens such as *Staphylococcusaureus* or *Bacillus cereus*, low numbers of bacteria can be cleared effectively by an adequate inflammatory response.[83] Once an inoculum threshold is passed, bacterial growth and toxin production overwhelm the inflammatory response. In an exhaustive attempt to clear the infection, PMN fill the posterior and anterior segments. Because the absence of TNFα has beendemonstrated to dampen the initial inflammatory response during *Bacillus cereus* endophthalmitis, several studies have also analyzed whether therapy targeting TNFα would effectively attenuate inflammation. The anti-inflammatory potential of anti-TNFα has been shown after injected immediately prior to *Bacillus cereus* infection.[82] Infliximab, anti-TNFα antibody has attenuated intraocular inflammation in experimental models of choroidal neovascularization, endotoxin-induced uveitis, and in human uveitis patients. [85-88] Infliximab was recently shown to be non-toxic at levels up to 1.7 mg in rabbit eyes. [89]

These findings suggest the potential for attenuation of inflammation during endophthalmitis by targeting TNFα and perhaps other cytokines, but this sort of therapy would likely be best suited for the initial stages of infection.[90] Continuing studies will determine the therapeutic potential of cytokine targeting in conjunction with early antibiotic treatment in reducing inflammation during endogenous endophthalmitis.

4. Future directions

Since AR has been advocated as an important therapeutic target to treat oxidative stress-induced inflammatory disorders including ocular inflammation, detailed studies of the molecular events and clear understanding of AR's involvement in the pathogenesis of inflammation is required. Understanding this role of AR should provide pharmacological tools for eventual therapeutic interventions to control cell proliferation, apoptosis, tissue repair, and prevention of the cytotoxicity of cytokines and chemokines which are elevated during ocular inflammation. More importantly, these studies will provide a mechanistic link between AR with ocular inflammation. Studies using various animal models are required to clearly understand the mechanism of AR's involvement in the inflammation and related pathologies which in turn will help in the design and synthesis of more specific inhibitors. Common limitations for some of the earlier AR inhibitors (ARI) such as sorbinil and tolrestat include critical hepatic and renal toxicity for long-term use. [91] Newer AR inhibitors such as zopolrestat, raneristat and fidarestat are now being tested for their ability to prevent the progression of diabetic neuropathy. Since these drugs have already passed in the Food and Drug Administration (FDA)'s phase I and II clinical trials and have been found to be safe without any major irreversible side effects, and it is expected that ARI such as fidarestat could be developed as novel therapy for preventing ocular inflammation especially uveitis in a relatively shorter time. [92-94]

Author details

Ozlem Sahin

Dunya Eye Hospital Ltd. Ankara, Turkey

References

[1] Mamalis N. Endophthalmitis. J Cataract Refract Surg. 2002;28(5):729–730.

[2] Essman TF, Flynn HW, Jr, Smiddy WE, et al. Treatment outcomes in a 10-year study of endogenous fungal endophthalmitis. Ophthalmic Surg Lasers. 1997;28(3):185–194.

[3] Jackson TL, Eykyn SJ, Graham EM, Stanford MR. Endogenous bacterial endophthalmitis: 17-year prospective series and review of 267 reported cases. Surg Ophthalmol. 2003;48(4):403–423.

[4] Okada AA, Johnson RP, Liles WC, D'Amico DJ, Baker AS. Endogenous bacterial endophthalmitis. Report of a ten-year retrospective study. Ophthalmology. 1994;101(5): 832–838.

[5] Rao NA, Hidayat AA. Endogenous mycotic endophthalmitis: Variations in clinical and histopathologic changes in candidiasis compared with aspergillosis. Am J Ophthalmol. 2001;132(2):244–251.

[6] Tanaka M, Kobayashi Y, Takebayashi H, Kiyokawa M, Qiu H. Analysis of predisposing clinical and laboratory findings for the development of endogenous fungal endophthalmitis. A retrospective 12-year study of 79 eyes of 46 patients. Retina. 2001;21(3):203–209.

[7] Kernt M, Kampik A. Endophthalmitis: pathogenesis, clinical presentation, management and prspectives. Clin Ophthalmol 2010;4:121-35.

[8] Dinani A, Ktaich N, Urban C, Rubin D.Levofloxacin-resistant-Streptococcus mitis endophthalmitis: a unique presentation of bacterial endocarditis.J Med Microbiol 2009;58:1385-7.

[9] Gery I, Streilein JW. Curr Opin Immunol. 1994;6:938–945.

[10] Forrester JV, McMenamin PG. Chem Immunol. 1999;73:159–185.

[11] Cho H, Wolf KJ, Wolf EJ. Clin Ophthalmol. 2009;3:199–210.

[12] Wagoner MD. Surv Ophthalmol. 1997;41:275–313.

[13] Cho H, Wolf KJ, Wolf EJ. Clin Ophthalmol. 2009;3:199–210.

[14] Mittag T. Exp Eye Res. 1984;39:759–769.

[15] Rao NA, Romero JL, Fernandez MA, Sevanian A, Marak GE., Jr Surv Ophthalmol. 1987;32:209–213.

[16] Rao NA. Trans Am Ophthalmol Soc. 1990;88:797–850.

[17] Ahn KS, Sethi G, Aggarwal BB. Curr Mol Med. 2007;7:619–637.

[18] Srivastava SK, Ramana KV. Exp Eye Res. 2009;88:2–3.

[19] Tak PP, Firestein GS. J Clin Invest. 2001;107:7–11

[20] Li Q, Verma IM. Nat Rev Immunol. 2002;2:725–734.

[21] Makarov SS. Mol Med Today. 2000;6:441–448.

[22] Uwe S. Biochem Pharmacol. 2008;75:1567–1579.

[23] Sarkar FH, Li Y, Wang Z, Kong D. Int Rev Immunol. 2008;27:293–319.

[24] Yadav UC, Srivastava SK, Ramana KV. Invest Ophthalmol Vis Sci. 2007;48:4634–4642.

[25] Pladzyk A, Reddy ABM, Yadav UCS, Tammali R, Ramana KV, Srivastava SK. Invest Ophthalmol Vis Sci. 2006;47:5395–5403.

[26] Ramana KV, Fadl AA, Tammali R, Reddy AB, Chopra AK, Srivastava SK. J Biol Chem. 2006;28:33019–33029.

[27] Pladzyk A, Reddy ABM, Yadav UCS, Tammali R, Ramana KV, Srivastava SK. Invest Ophthalmol Vis Sci. 2006;47:5395–5403.

[28] Akagi Y, Yajima Y, Kador PF, Kuwabara T, Kinoshita JH. Diabetes. 1984;33:562–566.

[29] Kinoshita JH, Kador P, Catiles M. JAMA. 1981;246:257–261.

[30] Streilein JW, Ohta K, Mo JS, Taylor AW. DNA Cell Biol. 2002;21:453–459.

[31] Yadav UC, Ighani-Hosseinabad F, van Kuijk FJ, Srivastava SK, Ramana KV. Invest Ophthalmol Vis Sci. 2009;50:752–759.

[32] Pladzyk A, Ramana KV, Ansari NH, Srivastava SK. Exp Eye Res. 2006;83:408–416.

[33] Yang P, de Vos AF, Kijlstra A. Br J Ophthalmol. 1997;81:396–401.

[34] McMenamin PG, Crewe J. Invest Ophthalmol Vis Sci. 1995;36:1949–1959.

[35] Kubo E, Urakami T, Fatma N, Akagi Y, Singh DP. Biochem Biophys Res Commun. 2004;314:1050–1056.

[36] Skeie JM, Mullins RF. Eye. 2009;23:747–755.

[37] Ohta K, Nakayama K, Kurokawa T, Kikuchi T, Yoshimura N. Invest Ophthalmol Vis Sci. 2002;43:744–750.

[38] De Rosa FG, Garazzino S, Pasero D, Di Perri G, Ranieri VM. Invasive candidiasis and candidemia: new guidelines. Minerva Anestesiol 2009;75:453-8.

[39] Weishaar PD, Flynn HW Jr, Murray TG, Davis JL, Barr JG, Mein CE, McLean WC Jr, Killian JH. Endogenous Aspergillus endophthalmitis. Clinical features and treatment outcomes. Ophthalmology 1988;105:57-65.

[40] Yonekawa Y, Chan RV, Reddy AK, Pieroni CG, Lee TC, Lee S. Early intravitreal treatment of endogenous bacterial endophthalmitis. Clin Experiment Ophthalmol 2011;39:771-8.

[41] Kain HL. Basic principles in the treatment of endophthalmitis. Klin Monbl Augenheilkd 1997;210:274-88.

[42] Meier P, Wiedemann P. Endophthalmitis: clinical Picture, therapy and prevention. Klin Monabl Augenheilkd 1997;210:175-91.

[43] Scoper SV. Review of third-and fourth-genertion fluoroquinolones in ophthal-mology:in-vitro and in-vivo efficay. Adv Ther 2008;25:979-94.

[44] Oliveria AD, D'Azevedo PA, Francisco W. In vitro activity of fluoroquinolones against ocular bacterial isolates in Sao Paulo, Brazil. Cornea 2007;26:194-8.

[45] Duggirala A, Joseph J, Sharma S, Nutheti R, Garg P, Das T. Activity of newer fluoroquinolones against gram-positive and gram-negative bascteria isolated from ocular infections: in vitro comparison. Indian J Ophthalmol 2007;55:15-9.

[46] Jackson TL, Eykyn SJ, Graham EM, Stanford MR. Endogenous bacterial endophthalmitis : a 17-year prospective series and review of 267 reported cases. Surv Ophthalmol 2003;48:403-23.

[47] Mather R, Karenchak LM, Romanowski EG, Kowalski RP. Fourth generation fluoroquinolones: new weapons in the Arsenal of ophthalmic antibiotics. Am J ophthalmol 2002;133:463-6.

[48] Oliveria AD, Höfling-Lima AL, Belfort R Jr, Gayoso Mde F, Francisco W. Fluoroquinolone susceptibilities to methicillin-resistant and susceptible coagulkase-negative Staphylococcus isolated from eye infection. Arq Bras Oftalmol 2007;70:286-9.

[49] Yagcı R, Oflu Y, Dinçel A, Kaya E, Yagcı S, Bayar B, Duman S, Bozkurt A. Penetration of second-third-and fourth generation topical fluoroquinolone into aqueous and vitreous humour in a rabbit endophthalmitis model. Eye 2007;21:990-4.

[50] Hariprasad SM, Shah GK, Chi J, Prince RA. Determination of aqueous and vitreous concentration of moxifloxacin 0.5% after delivery via a dissolvable corneal collagen shield device. J Cataract Refract Surg 2005;31:2142-6.

[51] Hariprasad SM, Mieler WF, Holz ER. Vitreous and aqueous penetration of orally administered gatifloxacin in humans. Arch Ophthalmol 2003;121:345-50.

[52] O'Brien TP. Besifloxacin ophthalmic suspension 0.6%: a novel topical fluoroquinolone for bacterial conjunctivitis. Adv Ther 2012; Epub ahead of print.

[53] Malhotra R, Gira J, Berdy GJ, Brusatti R. Safety of besifloxacin ophtahlmic suspension 0.6% as a prophylactic antibiotic following routine catarct surgery: result of a prospective, paralel-group, investigator-mascked study. Clin Ophtahlmol 2012;6:855-63.

[54] Donnenfeld ED, Comstock TL, Proksch JW. Human aqeous humor concentrations of besifloxacin, moxifloxacin, and gatifloxacin after topical ocular application. J Cataract Refract Surg 2011;37:1082-9.

[55] Norcross EW, Sanders ME, Moore Q 3rd, Sanfilippo CM, Hesje CK, Shafiee A, Marquart ME. Comparative efficacy of besifloxacin and other fluoroquinolones in a prophylaxis model of penicilin-resistant Streptococcus pneumoniae rabbit endophtahlmitis. Pharmacol Ther 201;26:237-43.

[56] Zhang JZ, Cavet ME, Ward KW. Anti-inflammatory effects of besiflocaxin, a novel fluoroquinolone, in primary human corneal epithelial cells. Curr Eye Res 2008;33:923-32.

[57] Wu X, Chen H, Jiang H, Xu Y, Liu T, Xu L. Prophylactic effect of topical fluoroquinolones in a rabbit model of Stapylococcus aureus endophthalmitis. J Ocul Pharmacol Ther 2012;28:186-93.

[58] Cornut PL, Chiquet C. Intravitreal injection of antibiotics in endophthalmitis. J Fr Ophthalmol 2008;31:815-23.

[59] Mehta S, Armstrong BK, Kim SJ, Toma H, West JN, Yin H, Lu P, Wayman LL, Recchia FM, Sternberg P Jr. Long-term potency, sterility, and stability of vancomycin, cftazidime, and moxifloxacin for traetment of bacterial endophthalmitis. Retina 2011;31:316-22.

[60] Shahar J, Zemel E, Perlman I, Loewenstein A. Physioloical and toxicological effects of cefuroxime on the albino rabbit retina. Invest Ophthalmol Vis Sci 2012;21:906-14.

[61] Yonekawa Y, Chan RV, Reddy AK, Pieroni CG, Lee TC, Lee S. Early intravitreal treatment of endogenous bacterial endophtahlmitis. Clin Experiment Ophthalmol 2011;39:771-8.

[62] Miller DM, Vedula AS, Flynn HW jr, Miller D, Scott WE, Murray TG, Venkatraman AS. Endophthalmitis caused by staphylococcus epidermidis: in vitro antibiotic susceptibilities and clinical outcomes. Ophthalmic Surg Lasers Imaging 2007;38:446-51.

[63] Albertcht E, Richards JC, Pollock T, Cook C, Myers L. Adjunctive use of intravitreal dexamethasone in presumed bacterial endophthalmitis: a randomised trial. Br J Ophthalmol 2011;95:385-8.

[64] Aslangul E, Le Jeunne C. Role of corticosteroids in infectious disease. Presse Med 2012;41:400-5.

[65] Liu F, Kwok AK, Cheung BM. The efficacy of intravitreal vancomycin and dexamethasone in the treatment of experimental bacillus cereus endophthalmitis. Curr Eye Res 2008;33:761-8.

[66] Jaffe GJ, McCallum RM, Branchaud B, Skalak C, Butuner Z, Ashton P. Long-term follow-up results of a pilot trial of a flucinolone acetonide implant to treat posterior uveitis. Ophthalmology 2005;112:1192-8.

[67] Chieh JJ, Crlson AN, Jaffe GJ. Combined flucinolone acetonide intraocular delivery system insertion, phacoemulsification and intraocular lens implantation for severe uveitis. Am J Ophthalmol 2008;146:589-94.

[68] Sarajya NV, Goldstein DA. DExamethasone for ocular inflammation. Expert Opin Pharmacother 2011;12:1127-31.

[69] Veritti D, Di Giulio A, Sarao V, Lanzetta P. Drug safety evaluation of intravitreal triamcinolone acetonide. Exp Opin Drug Saf 2012;11:331-40.

[70] Mulki L, Foster CS. Difluprednate for inflammatory eye disorders. Drugs Today (Barc) 2011;47:327-33.

[71] Essman TF, Flynn HW Jr, Smiddy WE, Brod RD, Murray TG, Davis JL, Rubsamen PE. Treatment outcomes in a 10-year study of endogenous fungal endophthalmitis. Ophthalmic Surg Lasers 1997;28:185-94.

[72] Weishaar PD, Flynn HW Jr, Murray TG, Davis JL, Barr CC, Gross JG, Mein CE, McLean WC Jr, Killian JH. Endogenous aspergillus endophthalmitis. Clinical features and treatment outcomes. Ophthalmology 1988;105:57-65.

[73] De Rosa FG, Garazzino S, pasero D, Di peri G, Ranieri VM. Invasive candidiasis and candidemia: new guidelines. Minerva Anestesiol 2009;75:453-8.

[74] Schulman JA, Peyman GA. Intravitreal corticosteroids as an adjunct in the traetment of bacterial and fungal endophthalmitis. A review. Retina 1992;12:336-40.

[75] Bazzoni F, Beutler B. The tumor necrosis factor ligand and receptor families. N Engl J Med. 1996;334:1717–25.

[76] Giese MJ, Sumner HL, Berliner JA, Mondino BJ. Cytokine expression in a rat model of Staphylococcus aureus endophthalmitis. Invest Ophthalmol Vis Sci. 1998;39:2785–90.

[77] Petropoulos IK, Vantzou CV, Lamari FN, Karamanos NK, Anastassiou ED, Pharmakakis NM. Expression of TNF-alpha, IL-1beta, and IFN-gamma in Staphylococcus epidermidis slime-positive experimental endophthalmitis is closely related to clinical inflammatory scores. Graefes Arch Clin Exp Ophthalmol. 2006;244:1322–28.

[78] Luna JD, Chan CC, Derevjanik NL, Mahlow J, Chiu C, Peng B, Tobe T, Campochiaro PA, Vinores SA. Blood-retinal barrier (BRB) breakdown in experimental autoimmune uveoretinitis: comparison with vascular endothelial growth factor, tumor necrosis factor alpha, and interleukin-1beta-mediated breakdown. J Neurosci Res. 1997;49:268–80.

[79] De Vos AF, Van Haren MA, Verhagen C, Hoekzema R, Kijlstra A. Tumour necrosis factor-induced uveitis in the Lewis rat is associated with intraocular interleukin 6 production. Exp Eye Res. 1995;60:199–207.

[80] Dick AD, Forrester JV, Liversidge J, Cope AP. The role of tumour necrosis factor (TNF-alpha) in experimental autoimmune uveoretinitis (EAU) Prog Retin Eye Res. 2004;23:617–37.

[81] Giese MJ, Rayner SA, Fardin B, Sumner HL, Rozengurt N, Mondino BJ, Gordon LK. Mitigation of neutrophil infiltration in a rat model of early Staphylococcus aureus endophthalmitis. Invest Ophthalmol Vis Sci. 2003;44:3077–82.

[82] Ramadan RT, Ramirez R, Novosad BD, Callegan MC. Acute inflammation and loss of retinal architecture and function during experimental Bacillus endophthalmitis. Curr Eye Res. 2006;31:955–65.

[83] Giese MJ, Sumner HL, Berliner JA, Mondino BJ. Cytokine expression in a rat model of Staphylococcus aureus endophthalmitis. Invest Ophthalmol Vis Sci. 1998;39:2785–90.

[84] Ravindranath RM, Hasan SA, Mondino BJ. Immunopathologic features of Staphylococcus epidermidis-induced endophthalmitis in the rat. Curr Eye Res. 1997;16:1036–43.

[85] Olson JL, Courtney RJ, Mandava N. Intravitreal infliximab and choroidal neovascularization in an animal model. Arch Ophthalmol. 2007;125:1221–24.

[86] Shi X, Semkova I, Müther PS, Dell S, Kociok N, Joussen AM. Inhibition of TNF-alpha reduces laser-induced choroidal neovascularization. Exp Eye Res. 2006;83:1325–34.

[87] Diaz-Llopis M, García-Delpech S, Salom D, Udaondo P, Bosch-Morell F, Quijada A, Romero FJ, Amselem L. High-dose infliximab prophylaxis in endotoxin-induced uveitis. J Ocul Pharmacol Ther. 2007;23:343–50.

[88] Gallagher M, Quinones K, Cervantes-Castañeda RA, Yilmaz T, Foster CS. Biological response modifier therapy for refractory childhood uveitis. Br J Ophthalmol. 2007;91:1341–44.

[89] Giansanti F, Ramazzotti M, Vannozzi L, Rapizzi E, Fiore T, Iaccheri B, Degl' Innocenti D, Moncini D, Menchini U. A pilot study on ocular safety of intravitreal infliximab in a rabbit model. Invest Ophthalmol Vis Sci. 2008;49:1151–56.

[90] Wiskur BW, Robinson M, Farrand A, Novosad B, Callegan MC. Improved therapeutic regimens for Bacillus endophthalmitis. Invest Ophthalmol Vis Sci. 2008;49:1480–87.

[91] Tsai SC, Burnakis TG. Aldose reductase inhibitors: an update. Ann Pharmacother 1993;27:751-4.

[92] Yadav UC, Shoeb M, Srivastava SK, Ramana KV. Aldose reductase deficiency protects from autoimmune- and endotoxin-induced uveitis in mice. Invest Ophthalmol Vis Sci 2011; 52:8076-85.

[93] Yadav UC, Shoeb M, Srivastava SK, Ramana KV. Amelioration of experimental autoimmune uveo-retinitis by aldose reductase inhibition in Lewis rats.Invest Ophthalmol Vis Sci 52:8033-41.

[94] Srivastava SK, Yadav UC, Reddy AB, Saxena A, Tammali R, Shoeb M, Ansari NH, Bhatnagar A, Petrash MJ, Srivastava S, Ramana KV. Aldose reductase inhibition suppresses oxidative stress-induced inflammatory disorders. Chem Biol Interact 2011;191:330-8.